Case Studies in Neuroscience

Case Studies in Neuroscience

Ralph F. Józefowicz, M.D.
Professor of Neurology and Medicine
Department of Neurology
University of Rochester
Rochester, New York

Robert G. Holloway, M.D., M.P.H.
Assistant Professor of Neurology and Community and Preventive Medicine
Department of Neurology
University of Rochester
Rochester, New York

F. A. Davis Company • Philadelphia

F. A. Davis Company
1915 Arch Street
Philadelphia, PA 19103

Printed in the United States of America

Last digit indicates print number: 10 9 8 7 6 5 4 3 2 1

Acquisitions Editor: Robert W. Reinhardt
Developmental Editor: Bernice M. Wissler
Production Editor: Elena Coler
Designer: Bill Donnelly
Cover Designer: Alicia Baronsky
Cover Art: Ryoko Oda, Perkins and Will, New York, NY, by permission of the University of Rochester School of Medicine and Dentistry.
Illustrator: Kurt Pakan

As new scientific information becomes available through basic and clinical research, recommended treatments and drug therapies undergo changes. The author(s) and publisher have done everything possible to make this book accurate, up to date, and in accord with accepted standards at the time of publication. The authors, editors, and publisher are not responsible for errors or omissions or for consequences from application of the book, and make no warranty, expressed or implied, in regard to the contents of the book. Any practice described in this book should be applied by the reader in accordance with professional standards of care used in regard to the unique circumstances that may apply in each situation. The reader is advised always to check product information (package inserts) for changes and new information regarding dose and contraindications before administering any drug. Caution is especially urged when using new or infrequently ordered drugs.

Library of Congress Cataloging-in-Publication Data

Józefowicz, Ralph F., 1953-
    Case studies in neuroscience / Ralph F. Józefowicz, Robert G. Holloway.
    p.   cm.
    Includes index.
    ISBN 0-8036-0304-5
    1. Nervous system—Diseases—Case studies.   2. Neuroanatomy—Case studies.   3. Neurophysiology—Case studies.   I. Holloway, Robert G., 1963- . II. Title.
    RC359.J69   1000
    616.8—dc21   98-48503
                                                                                                CIP

Preface

This book is an outgrowth of the case study syllabus used at the University of Rochester for the first-year medical student Neural Science course. These 27 case studies are felt to be the most successful part of the Neural Science course and form the backbone of the small-group sessions of this course.

Although these cases contain much clinical information, the point of these clinical case studies is to learn neuroanatomy and neurophysiology; a knowledge of clinical neurology is not necessary to work through them. In fact, key clinical neurologic terms are defined at the beginning of each case.

This book is primarily intended for use by preclinical medical students in an integrated Neural Science course. It should also prove extremely useful for students in a neurology clerkship, residents rotating on neurology, and nursing and physical therapy student studying neurology.

The cases contained in this book were written by many neurology residents and faculty, including Curtis Benesch, James Gaffney, Daniel Giang, Karl Kieburtz, Seth Kolkin, Louis Medved, Heidi Schwarz, and James Wymer, and have been extensively revised based on student feedback. We would like to thank these individuals as well as the medical students and neurology residents at the University of Rochester for their help in writing and revising these cases. We also wish to thank Kurt Pakan for the illustrations that accompany the answers.

Ralph F. Józefowicz, MD
Robert G. Holloway, MD, MPH
Rochester, New York

v

Contents

These 27 clinical case studies were prepared to illustrate the crucial application of the basic neural sciences to problems in clinical neurology. Each case illustrates a specific section of regional or systemic neuroanatomy and many are accompanies by computed tomography or magnetic resonance images of the nervous system.

To benefit the most from each case, prepare beforehand by reading the case carefully, studying the key words, and trying to answer the questions. You may find several of the standard clinical neurology textbooks helpful in this regard. After you have answered the questions yourself, you should then (and only then) compare your answers with the "correct" answers, which may be found at the end of each case.

Remember that the purpose of these cases is not to "guess the diagnosis" but to gain a better understanding of neuroanatomy and neurophysiology as they apply to clinical neurology. Although it is not our primary intent to teach you clinical neurology through these case studies, we strongly feel that by stressing the clinical applications of basic neurosciences, you will not only better appreciate the relevance of the basic neurosciences to clinical neurology, but also learn these disciplines more thoroughly and effectively.

The Clumsy Graduate Student

Case 1

KEY TERMS

upper motor neuron: A neuron whose cell body lies in the motor area of the cerebral cortex or in certain brain stem nuclei (red nucleus, lateral and medial vestibular nuclei, pontine and medullary reticular formations, superior and inferior colliculi).

lower motor neuron: A neuron whose cell body lies in the anterior gray column of the spinal cord or in certain cranial nerve motor nuclei (oculomotor, abducens, trigeminal motor, trochlear, facial, ambiguus, hypoglossal).

miosis: Abnormal contraction of the pupils, possibly due to irritation of the oculomotor system or paralysis of dilators.

ptosis: Drooping of the upper eyelid due to paralysis of the levator palpebrae or superior tarsal muscles.

sensory level: A horizontal level on the trunk corresponding to a specific strip of skin innervated by a particular spinal cord segment, below which there is a loss or diminution of sensations owing to a lesion of the spinal cord.

proprioception: The awareness of posture, movement, and changes in equilibrium and the knowledge of position, weight, and resistance of objects in relation to the body.

plantar response: Movement of the great toe in response to plantar stimulation with a noxious stimulus. Flexion of the great toe is a normal response; extension of the great toe implies upper motor neuron pathology and is known as Babinski's sign.

magnetic resonance (MR) scan: A method of imaging the body that utilizes the nuclear magnetic resonance properties of the hydrogen ion and results in a water-fat tissue density ratio that is converted by computer analysis into an image.

autonomic nervous system: The part of the nervous system that controls involuntary bodily functions

sympathetic nervous system: The thoracolumbar division of the autonomic nervous system.

visual evoked responses (VER): A method for measuring the conduction velocity in the optic nerve by summating the scalp electric potentials from the occipital lobe, which are elicited in response to a series of patterned visual stimuli.

HISTORY AND EXAMINATION

History of the Present Illness

A 24-year-old, right-handed graduate student presents to the emergency room because of left arm clumsiness. Five days previously, she noted difficulty performing fine motor movements with her left hand, particularly when buttoning her blouse. Over the ensuing 5 days, her symptoms gradually worsened, and now her entire left arm feels weak and clumsy. Occasionally, she experiences a sharp pain starting in her neck and radiating down her left arm into her left thumb. For the past 24 hours, she has felt unsteady on her feet and thinks this may be related to a clumsy left leg. She also reports an abnormal sensation in her right leg. For example, hot bath water does not feel as "hot" with her right leg as compared with her left. She also describes an electric "shocklike" sensation radiating down her spine whenever she flexes her neck forward. She reports no bladder difficulties, headache, diplopia, or vertigo.

Past Medical History

Unremarkable

Medications

Birth control pills

Physical Examination

She appears well and has the following vital signs: BP = 118/56 mm Hg; P = 68/min; R = 12/min; T = 36.9°C. Her neck has full range of motion.

Neurological Examination

Her mental status is intact. There is mild left ptosis. Her pupils are (R/L) 6/4.5 mm reacting briskly to 3/2.5 mm. Her fundi reveal sharp, flat discs. Ocular motility is full, without nystagmus. Facial strength is normal. Corneal reflexes and facial sensation are intact bilaterally. There is increased tone in the left arm and leg. Functional strength testing is normal and formal muscle power is as follows (R/L): deltoid 5/4, biceps 5/4, triceps 5/4+, wrist extensors 5/4-, wrist flexors 5/4-, hand intrinsics 5/3-, hip flexors 5/4+, all other groups 5/5. Her fine motor movements with her left hand are impaired. She has decreased pinprick and temperature sensation on the right leg and right trunk to about T2. Proprioception and vibratory sensation are mildly decreased on her left leg compared with the right. Muscle stretch reflexes are increased on the left compared with the right, and her left plantar response is extensor. Abdominal reflexes are absent on the left. Her gait was not tested.

She was sent for an emergent MR scan that evening.

Questions

1. What is a dissociated sensory loss? List three conditions that result in a dissociated sensory loss. Does this patient have a dissociated sensory loss?

2. What do you call the electric shocklike sensation she experiences when she flexes her neck? In what neurological disorders is this sign commonly seen?

3. What is miosis? Does this patient have miosis? What is the triad of ptosis, miosis, and anhidrosis called? List all the possible levels of the neuraxis at which a lesion can produce this triad. Why does this patient have ptosis?

4. The eyelid is elevated by two different muscles supplied by two different nerves. Name these muscles, their innervation, and describe their functions. Can you differentiate between the two on clinical examination? Which one do you think is affected in this patient?

5. Why are her left arm and leg clumsy?

6. What is a plantar response, and why is the left plantar response extensor?

7. What are abdominal reflexes? What is the significance of the abdominal reflex asymmetry in this patient?

8. Identify the one neuroanatomic region in this patient that, if lesioned, can explain all of her symptoms. What is the name given to this symptom complex?

9. MR scans of her cervical spine are shown in Figure 1. What abnormality do you see? What is your differential diagnosis of this woman's problem? What is the most likely diagnosis?

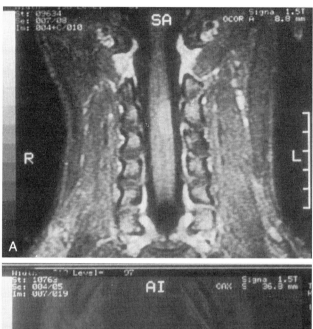

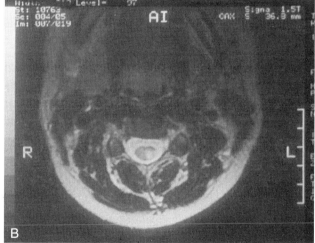

Figure 1. *(A)* T1-weighted coronal MR scan of the cervical spine with gadolinium. *(B)* T2-weighted axial image of the cervical spine.

10. What further diagnostic tests would you consider at this point? What treatment would you recommend?

Answers

1. What is a dissociated sensory loss? List three conditions that result in a dissociated sensory loss. Does this patient have a dissociated sensory loss?

    Dissociated sensory loss: A regional sensory loss that involves only one of the two primary sensory modalities, with sparing of the other, that is, loss of pain and temperature perception (small fiber—spinothalamic system) with sparing of vibratory sensation and proprioception (large fiber—dorsal column system) or vice versa. There are two different situations in which this type of sensory loss may occur:
    - A brain stem or spinal cord lesion that affects either the spinothalamic system or the dorsal column system.
    - A peripheral neuropathy that selectively involves only small, unmyelinated sensory fibers or large, myelinated sensory fibers.

    Conditions that may produce a dissociated sensory loss include:
    - Lateral medullary syndrome (brain stem stroke)
    - Syringomyelia (central cavitation of the spinal cord)
    - Brown-Séquard's syndrome ("hemisection" of the spinal cord)
    - Axonal neuropathy, affecting small, unmyelinated fibers only
    - Demyelinating neuropathy, affecting large, myelinated fibers only

    This patient demonstrates a dissociated sensory loss in which spinothalamic function is impaired on her right, and dorsal column function is impaired on her left.

2. What do you call the electric shocklike sensation she experiences when she flexes her neck? In what neurological disorders is this sign commonly seen?

    Lhermitte's sign: A sudden electric-like or painful sensation spreading down the body or into the back or extremities with flexion of the neck. This sign can be seen with any lesion to the cervical spinal cord, including demyelination as in multiple sclerosis (MS), tumor, herniated disc, or a bony ridge indenting the cord.

3. What is miosis? Does this patient have miosis? What is the triad of ptosis, miosis, and anhidrosis called? List all the possible levels of the neuraxis at which a lesion can produce this triad. Why does this patient have ptosis?

Miosis: A unilateral constricted pupil. This patient has left-sided miosis.

Horner's syndrome: A clinical triad consisting of ptosis, miosis, and (at times) anhidrosis (dry skin due to an inability to perspire), which is caused by a lesion to the sympathetic nerve fibers that innervate the face (Fig. 2). The sympathetic nervous system, along with the parasympathetic nervous system, makes up the autonomic nervous system, which controls many involuntary body functions.

Horner's syndrome may be caused by an ipsilateral lesion in the hypothalamus, brain stem reticular formation, cervical and upper thoracic spinal cord, superior cervical ganglion, or sympathetic fibers running along the carotid artery and the branches of cranial nerve V.

The most likely cause of ptosis (and miosis) in this patient is a lesion involving the lower cervical and upper thoracic spinal cord. The reason for this is that she also has left upper extremity weakness and a "sensory level" at T2 (a spinal cord level below which sensation is abnormal). The only location along the neuraxis where a single lesion may result in these signs is the lower cervical and upper thoracic spinal cord. Furthermore, she has no clinical evidence for hypothalamic or brain stem dysfunction.

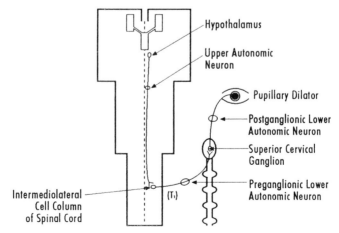

Figure 2. Sympathetic nervous system.

4. The eyelid is elevated by two different muscles supplied by two different nerves. Name these muscles, their innervation, and describe their functions. Can you differentiate between the two on clinical examination? Which one do you think is affected in this patient?

Levator palpebrae: Skeletal muscle innervated by cranial nerve III whose function is voluntary lid elevation.

Superior tarsal muscle (also known as Müller's muscle): Smooth muscle innervated by the sympathetic nervous system, and under involuntary control.

One can distinguish which muscle is involved in a patient with ptosis by having the patient voluntarily look up. With voluntary upward gaze, ptosis due to sympathetic dysfunction resolves, indicating that the superior tarsal muscle is involved. In this patient, the ptosis is most likely due to involvement of the sympathetic nervous system as part of Horner's syndrome.

5. Why are her left arm and leg clumsy?

This patient has left leg hyperreflexia and increased muscle tone in the left limbs as well as a left plantar extensor response. All these signs are suggestive of upper motor neuron dysfunction, most probably due to an ipsilateral lesion affecting the left corticospinal tract in the cervical or thoracic spinal cord. She also has reduced vibratory perception and proprioception (position sense) in the left leg, suggesting involvement of the dorsal column sensory system, most probably due to an ipsilateral lesion affecting the left fasciculus gracilis in the cervical or thoracic spinal cord.

6. What is a plantar response, and why is the left plantar response extensor?

Plantar response: A superficial, nociceptive reflex elicited by stroking the lateral plantar surface of the foot from the heel toward the ball of the foot. The normal response is plantar flexion of the great toe. Extension of the great toe implies an upper motor neuron lesion and is known as Babinski's sign. A lesion involving the corticospinal tract at any level of the neuraxis may result in an extensor plantar response.

Theoretically, a lesion at any level of the neuraxis may account for the left plantar extensor response. However, a lesion involving the lower cervical and upper thoracic spinal cord, accounting for her left arm and leg clumsiness (discussed in question No. 5), is the most likely explanation in this case.

7. What are abdominal reflexes? What is the significance of the abdominal reflex asymmetry in this patient?

   Abdominal reflexes: Superficial, nociceptive reflexes obtained by stroking the skin lightly on the abdomen from the umbilicus toward any abdominal quadrant and observing for deviation of the umbilicus toward the quadrant that is stroked. Absence of abdominal reflexes on one side suggests upper motor neuron dysfunction and is roughly equivalent to an extensor plantar response (Babinski's sign).

   The asymmetry in this patient suggests ipsilateral upper motor neuron dysfunction.

8. Identify the one neuroanatomic region in this patient that, if lesioned, can explain all of her symptoms. What is the name given to this symptom complex?

   A lesion in the left cervical spinal cord can produce ipsilateral upper motor neuron dysfunction, ipsilateral dorsal column sensory dysfunction, and contralateral spinothalamic sensory dysfunction. This symptom complex is referred to as *Brown-Séquard's syndrome* (hemisection of the spinal cord) (Fig. 3). This lesion can also explain the additional neurological findings in this patient, including the ipsilateral Horner's syndrome, cervical radicular (nerve root) pain, and Lhermitte's sign.

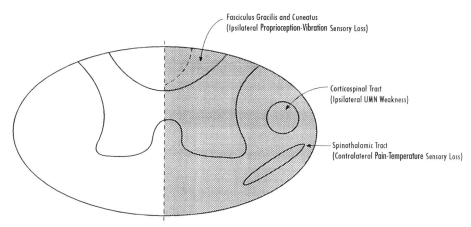

Figure 3. Brown-Séquard's syndrome. UMN = upper motor neuron.

9. MR scans of her cervical spine are shown in Figure 1. What abnormality do you see? What is your differential diagnosis of this woman's problem? What is the most likely diagnosis?

The scans show an intramedullary lesion in the left midcervical spinal cord (shown on the right side of the figure), extending from C3 to approximately C5. The lesion is remarkably confined to the left half of the cervical spinal cord and appears as a high-signal (bright) area in the shape of a semicircle. The lesion demonstrated minimal contrast enhancement with gadolinium (images not shown).

The differential diagnosis of this focal spinal cord signal abnormality includes myelitis due to either demyelinating disease, an infection, or vasculitis. The differential diagnosis also includes low-grade tumor (e.g., astrocytoma), although this is unlikely, given the acuity of her symptoms.

The most likely diagnosis for this condition is a demyelinating process, given the patient's age and the lack of risk factors for infection or vasculitis. This demyelinating lesion might be the first manifestation of MS in this patient.

10. What further diagnostic tests would you consider at this point? What treatment would you recommend?

The main reason to perform additional diagnostic procedures in this patient is to look for additional demyelinating lesions or evidence of central nervous system (CNS) immunoglobulin synthesis, both of which would suggest a diagnosis of MS. These tests include:

- **Head MR scan,** looking for additional demyelinating lesions suggestive of MS.
- **Visual evoked responses,** a measure of conduction velocity in the optic nerve. Demyelinating lesions due to MS in the optic nerve (a nerve tract in the CNS) should produce slowing in conduction velocity in this nerve.
- **Lumbar puncture,** looking for oligoclonal bands. Their presence indicates local immunoglobulin synthesis in the CNS, which is highly suggestive of MS.

Treatment

If no infectious source is identified, a course of intravenous steroids should be considered for symptomatic treatment of the patient's neurological symptoms. Corticosteroids help suppress the inflammatory component of demyelination and speed clinical and pathologic recovery from an episode of demyelination.

If the diagnosis of multiple sclerosis is substantiated by finding additional demyelinating lesions, either on VER testing or on the head MR scan, then the patient should be considered for prophylactic therapy to reduce the frequency of future exacerbations. Presently available prophylactic agents include the β-interferons and glatiramer acetate (Copaxone).

The Burned
Barbecue Chef

KEY TERMS

hand intrinsic muscles: A muscle that has both its origin and insertion within the hand.

muscle stretch reflexes: An involuntary muscle contraction that follows rapid passive stretch of a muscle spindle evoked by striking the attached tendon with a percussion hammer; deep tendon reflex.

dissociated sensory loss: A pattern of cutaneous sensory loss in which only one of the two primary sensory modalities (pain and temperature or vibration and proprioception) is affected in a specific body region.

spastic catch: A velocity-dependent resistance to passive stretch of a muscle that immediately relaxes and "gives way."

atrophy: A wasting or decrease in size of skeletal muscle, usually due to denervation or disuse; to undergo or cause atrophy.

central nervous system: The brain and spinal cord.

syrinx: A pathologic cavity in the spinal cord or brain.

HISTORY AND EXAMINATION

History of the Present Illness

A 42-year-old, right-handed man presents to your office after he accidentally burned his left hand. Four days previously, he was tending the grill at his company's summer barbecue. He repeatedly checked if the charcoal was ready by holding his left hand above the briquettes. Although the briquettes had a searing glow, he discovered that he could not appreciate their hot temperature with his left hand. In fact, he subsequently developed second-degree burns over his left forearm. This prompted him to seek medical attention.

The patient denies ever having had previous sensory symptoms. When specifically questioned, he agrees with you that both of his hands have lost muscle bulk but claims that they have been that way for years. Occasionally, he experiences right neck pain that radiates down his right arm and which he describes as burning in quality. Otherwise, he reports no other symptoms.

Past Medical History

Appendectomy

Medications

None

Physical Examination

He has mild kyphoscoliosis. Neck and shoulder range of motion is normal.

Neurological Examination

Mental status and cranial nerve examinations are normal. On motor examination, there is decreased muscle bulk in the hand intrinsic muscles bilaterally and in the left forearm. A mild spastic catch is present in both legs. Formal strength testing reveals the following (R/L): deltoids 5/5, biceps 5/5, triceps 5/5, wrist extensors 5-/4+, wrist flexors 4+/4+, hand intrinsics 4/4-. Lower extremity strength is normal bilaterally. On sensory testing, he has loss of thermal sense and pinprick over the posterior neck and shoulders and extending down both arms in a "capelike" fashion. Muscle stretch reflexes reveal the following (R/L): biceps 1/1, triceps 0/0, brachioradialis 1/1, knee jerks 3/3, ankle jerks 3/3. The plantar response is extensor on the right and flexor on the left. His gait is normal, other than for mild difficulty with tandem walking.

After your initial evaluation, you send him for an additional diagnostic test.

Questions

1. Detail the proprioception-vibration and pain-temperature sensory pathways that subserve the arms. Where do they cross in the neuraxis?

2. Is the weakness in the patient's arms due to lower motor neuron or upper motor neuron dysfunction? Why?

3. Is a dissociated sensory loss present in this case? If so, how does it differ from that in case 1?

4. How do you explain the fact that the patient burned his left forearm but never complained of left arm numbness?

5. Why does the patient have spasticity in his legs and a plantar extensor response on the right?

6. Why does the patient have atrophy of the intrinsic hand muscles?

7. Can a lesion in one neuroanatomic region explain the patient's neurological findings? How does this case differ from case 1?

8. Figure 4 is the T1-weighted sagittal magnetic resonance (MR) scan that you ordered. What does it show?

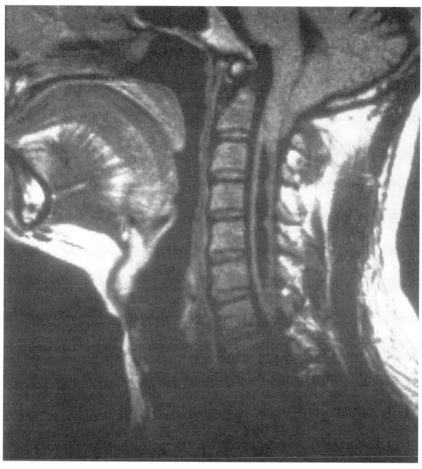

Figure 4. T1-weighted sagittal MR scan of the cervical spine.

9. Figure 5 shows a pathologic specimen from a patient with a similar condition (but who died of other causes). Explain in neuroanatomic detail how this condition could explain all of the patient's symptoms.

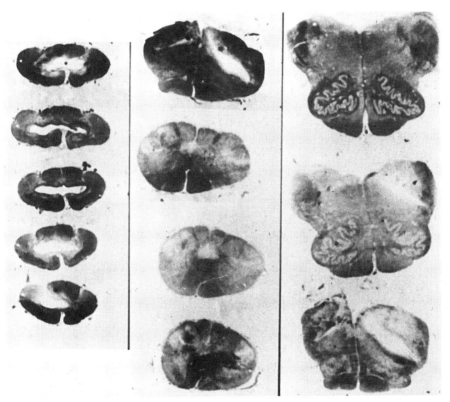

Figure 5. Myelin stain of the spinal cord and medulla.

10. Can other pathologic states lead to a similar clinical syndrome? If so, what are they?

11. What treatments are available for this patient?

Answers

1. Detail the proprioception-vibration and pain-temperature sensory pathways that subserve the arms. Where do they cross in the neuraxis?

Proprioception-Vibration Pathways

The primary sensory neurons begin as encapsulated nerve endings, with the cell bodies located in the dorsal root ganglia (Fig. 6). The proximal portions of the axons of these neurons then enter the spinal cord via the dorsal roots and project cephalad in the dorsal columns to the gracilis and cuneate nuclei of the medulla, synapsing on secondary sensory neurons in these nuclei. Axons from these nuclei cross the midline as the internal arcuate fibers of the medulla and ascend in the medial lemniscus, synapsing on tertiary sensory neurons located in nucleus ventralis posterolateral (VPL) of the thalamus. These tertiary sensory axons then project to the primary sensory cortex in the postcentral gyrus.

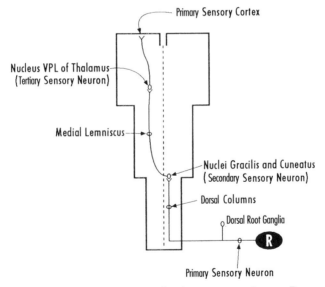

Figure 6. The proprioception-vibration sensory pathways. R = receptor, VPL = ventral posterolateral.

Pain-Temperature Pathways

- **Fast pain and temperature:** The primary sensory neurons begin as small myelinated fibers (Aδ fibers) with their cell bodies located in the dorsal root ganglia (Fig. 7). The proxi-

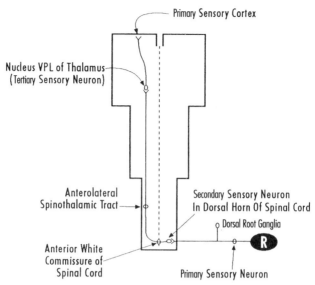

Figure 7. The fast pain and temperature sensory pathways. R = receptor, VPL = ventral posterolateral.

mal portions of the axons of these neurons then enter the spinal cord via the dorsal roots and synapse on secondary sensory neurons located in the dorsal horn of the spinal cord. Axons from these secondary sensory neurons cross the midline in the anterior white commissure of the spinal cord and ascend in the contralateral spinothalamic tract up through the brain stem, finally synapsing on tertiary sensory neurons located in nucleus VPL of the thalamus. These tertiary sensory axons then project to the primary sensory cortex in the post-central gyrus.

• **Slow pain:** The primary sensory neurons begin as bare nerve endings (C fibers) with their cell bodies located in the dorsal root ganglia (Fig. 8). The proximal portions of the axons of these neurons then enter the spinal cord via the dorsal roots and synapse on secondary sensory neurons located in the dorsal horn of the spinal cord. Axons from these secondary sensory neurons cross the midline in the anterior white commissure of the spinal cord and ascend in the contralateral spinothalamic and spinoreticular tracts up through the brain stem, finally synapsing on tertiary sensory neurons located in the centromedian nucleus of the thalamus. These tertiary sensory axons then project to the secondary sensory cortex.

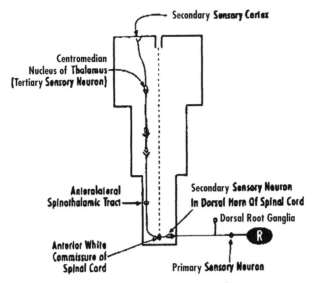

Figure 8. The slow pain sensory pathways. R = receptor.

2. Is the weakness in the patient's arms due to lower motor neuron or upper motor neuron dysfunction? Why?

   It is due to *lower motor neuron dysfunction,* because of the associated decreased muscle bulk and hypoactive muscle stretch reflexes. In upper motor neuron dysfunction, one would expect muscle bulk to be preserved and muscle stretch reflexes to be hyperactive. One would also expect the plantar response to be extensor with upper motor neuron lesions.

3. Is a dissociated sensory loss present in this case? If so, how does it differ from that in case 1?

   Yes, a dissociated sensory loss is present in this case. It differs from the first case both in the pattern of sensory loss and in the location of the lesion. In case 1 the spinothalamic tract and dorsal column system are lesioned on one side of the cervical spinal cord, producing ipsilateral loss of vibratory perception and proprioception, and contralateral loss of pain and temperature sensation; the other side of the spinal cord remains intact. In this case, this patient has bilateral pain and temperature sensory dysfunction in the upper extremities and upper back, with sparing of vibration and proprioception sensory function. The most likely cause is a lesion to the anterior white commissure of the cervical spinal cord in the midline, because this is the only place where a single lesion can affect both right and left pain-temperature pathways.

4. How do you explain the fact that the patient burned his left forearm but never complained of left arm numbness?

Since his vibration and proprioception sensation remains intact, he does not note numbness.

5. Why does the patient have spasticity in his legs and a plantar extensor response on the right?

Most likely he has involvement of both right and left corticospinal tracts in the spinal cord, with the right one being more affected than the left (and thus producing a right plantar extensor response). One type of lesion affecting both corticospinal tracts (as well as the anterior white commissure) is a central cervical syrinx (central cavitation of the spinal cord), which may cause outward compressive effects on the descending corticospinal tracts located in the lateral funiculi.

6. Why does the patient have atrophy of the intrinsic hand muscles?

He most likely has damage to the lower motor neurons in the ventral horns of the cervical spinal cord.

7. Can a lesion in one neuroanatomic region explain the patient's neurological findings? How does this case differ from case 1?

A *central* lesion in the cervical spinal cord, such as a syrinx, can account for all of the patient's neurological findings. By encroaching on nuclei and tracts located in the central portion of the cervical spinal cord, a syrinx can explain all of this patient's signs and symptoms as follows:

Symptom or Sign	Structure Affected in the Central Cervical Spinal Cord
Intrinsic hand muscle atrophy	Anterior horn cells in the ventral horns
Hand and wrist muscle weakness	Anterior horn cells in the ventral horns
Upper extremity hyporeflexia	Anterior horn cells in the ventral horns
Pain-temperature sensory loss in a capelike distribution	Anterior white commissure
Leg spasticity and hyperreflexia	Corticospinal tracts
Right plantar extensor response	Right corticospinal tract

In contrast, the lesion in case 1 involves the entire left lateral cervical spinal cord.

8. Figure 4 is the T1-weighted sagittal MR scan that you ordered. What does it show?

It shows a hypodense or dark area in the center of the spinal cord, extending from C1 to C5. This central cavity of cerebrospinal fluid density in the cervical spinal cord is consistent with a syrinx. Although the fourth ventricle appears relatively normal, there is mild downward herniation of the cerebellar tonsils, which are seen in the upper posterior spinal canal.

9. Figure 5 shows a pathologic specimen from a patient with a similar condition (but who died of other causes). Explain in neuroanatomic detail how this condition could explain all of the patient's symptoms.

Figure 5 shows a series of cross-sectional pathologic specimens revealing a cystic cavitation of the central portion of the cervical spinal cord and lower medulla. As the syrinx enlarges, it may compress and destroy the anterior white commissure, anterior horns, and lateral funiculi.

A dissociated segmental anesthesia over the neck, shoulders, and arms (capelike distribution) is caused by damage to the crossing anterior white commissure fibers. The weakness and atrophy of the hands and arms with loss of upper extremity muscle stretch reflexes represent damage to the anterior horn cells in the ventral horns of the spinal cord. The upper motor neuron signs in the lower extremities (hyperreflexia and spasticity as well as the right plantar extensor response) are due to damage to the descending corticospinal tracts in the lateral funiculi.

10. Can other pathologic states lead to a similar clinical syndrome? If so, what are they?

The syringomyelic syndrome is most often due to syringomyelia (a central cavitation of the spinal cord), but a similar clinical syndrome may sometimes be observed in association with other pathologic states. These include intramedullary spinal cord tumors, traumatic myelopathy ("myelo" refers to the spinal cord), postradiation myelopathy, spinal arachnoiditis, spinal cord infarction, and bleeding into the spinal cord (hematomyelia).

11. What treatments are available for this patient?

Limited therapy is available for patients with syringomyelia. One therapeutic option is a syringostomy, which involves shunting the fluid in the cavity into the subarachnoid space. Unfortunately, this neurosurgical procedure is risky, and the long-term benefit is unpredictable.

The Sidelined Billiard Champion

KEY TERMS

dermatome: A delineated area of skin innervated by a spinal cord segment.

segmental sensory loss: Sensory loss in the distribution of a dermatome.

clonus: Spasmodic alternation of muscular contractions between antagonistic muscle groups caused by a hyperactive stretch reflex from an upper motor neuron lesion.

hyperreflexia: An increased action of the reflexes.

spasticity: Increased tone or contractions of muscles causing stiff and awkward movements; the result of an upper motor neuron lesion.

Valsalva's maneuver: An attempt to forcibly exhale with the glottis, nose, and mouth closed.

urinary urgency: A sudden, almost uncontrollable need to urinate.

paresthesia: A sensation of numbness, prickling, or tingling; heightened sensitivity; experienced in central and peripheral nerve lesions.

HISTORY AND EXAMINATION

History of the Present Illness

A 41-year-old, left-handed billiard champion presents to your office with left neck pain and left arm weakness. He recently completed his U.S. tour and experienced increasing left neck and arm pain over the past 6 weeks. He describes it as a lancinating pain that radiates down the radial aspect of his left forearm. He also notes paresthesias of the left thumb and index finger. The pain is precipitated by pulling back the billiard stick with his left arm when shooting billiards, a symptom he believes caused his recent tour defeat. In addition, the pain is aggravated when he sneezes. He also feels that his left arm is slightly weak, and he found it more difficult to carry his luggage with his left arm at the end of the tour. Over the past week, he feels that his walking has been a bit unsteady. He also has a sense of urgency when he needs to urinate. This urgency was not present 1 week ago.

Past Medical History

Chronic low-back pain

Medications

Naprosyn for low-back pain

Physical Examination

The patient is in mild discomfort and reluctant to move his neck in any direction. BP = 130/74 mm Hg; P = 76/min. He has excellent shoulder and elbow range of motion.

Neurological Examination

The patient's mental status and cranial nerves are normal. On motor testing, he has mild spasticity in the lower extremities with clonus at the ankles bilaterally. Formal strength testing reveals the following (R/L): deltoids 5/5, biceps 5/4+, triceps 5/5, wrist extensors 5/5. Lower extremity strength is normal bilaterally. He has no ataxia. On sensory examination, there is decreased pinprick perception over the lateral aspect of his entire left arm extending down to his left thumb and second digit. There is no truncal sensory level. Muscle stretch reflexes are as follows (R/L): triceps 3/3, biceps 2/0, brachioradialis 2/0, knee 3+/3+, ankle 4/4. Plantar responses are extensor bilaterally. Casual gait is normal, but he does have some difficulty with tandem walking.

Questions

1. Sensory loss could be due to a lesion involving a peripheral nerve, nerve root, spinal cord or brain stem, thalamus, or cortical sensory areas. How do the patient's sensory examination findings help differentiate among these various lesions? Explain your answer.

2. Do you think that the patient's left arm weakness is due to lower motor neuron or upper motor neuron dysfunction? Explain your answer.

3. Why do you think that the patient is complaining of gait unsteadiness and difficulty with tandem walking?

4. Why is the pain aggravated when he sneezes?

5. Why is he complaining of urinary urgency?

6. What is meant by a truncal sensory level? Why is it important to look for this pattern of sensory loss in this patient?

7. Why are his triceps muscle stretch reflexes hyperactive?

8. Can a lesion in one neuroanatomic region explain all of the patient's neurological findings? Account for all of the motor, sensory, and autonomic symptoms.

9. Explain in detail how one lesion could produce lower motor neuron signs in the upper extremities and upper motor neuron signs in the lower extremities?

10. Figure 9 shows sagittal and axial cervical magnetic resonance (MR) scans obtained on admission. What is your diagnosis?

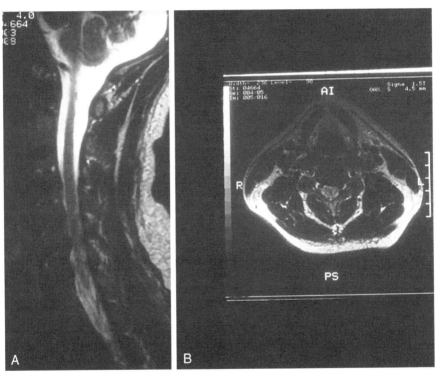

Figure 9. *(A)* T2-weighted sagittal cervical MR scan. *(B)* T2-weighted axial cervical MR scan.

11. What different forms of treatment are available for this patient, and what would you recommend?

Answers

1. Sensory loss could be due to a lesion involving a peripheral nerve, nerve root, spinal cord or brain stem, thalamus, or cortical sensory areas. How do the patient's sensory examination findings help differentiate among these various lesions? Explain your answer.

   The sensory loss seen in this patient (lateral aspect of the left arm extending into the left thumb and second digit) conforms to the sensory distribution of the left C6 nerve root (left C6 dermatome) and is most likely due to a lesion involving this nerve root. A dermatome is a strip of skin supplied by an individual spinal nerve (a nerve root).

   Lesions to peripheral nerves, spinal cord, or more rostral sensory areas produce different patterns of sensory loss. For example, a spinal cord lesion may produce a sensory level, below which sensation is impaired. A lesion in the brain stem or more rostral areas may produce a sensory loss on only one side of the body (a hemisensory loss).

2. Do you think the patient's left arm weakness is due to lower motor neuron or upper motor neuron dysfunction? Explain your answer.

   The patient's left arm weakness is due to lower motor neuron (LMN) dysfunction, because of the left biceps weakness associated with absent left biceps and brachioradialis muscle stretch reflexes.

   An upper motor neuron (UMN) lesion would produce hyperactive upper extremity muscle stretch reflexes.

3. Why do you think that the patient is complaining of gait unsteadiness and difficulty with tandem walking?

   Most likely these symptoms are due to UMN dysfunction, because of the patient's hyperreflexic knee and ankle muscle stretch reflexes and his bilateral plantar extensor responses. The most likely explanation for the UMN signs in this patient is a lesion to the corticospinal tracts in the cervical spinal cord, because evidence already exists of cervical nerve root lesion.

   This table summarizes the different motor findings in patients with UMN and LMN lesions:

Finding	UMN Lesion	LMN Lesion
Muscle bulk	Preserved	Atrophy
Muscle tone	Spastic	Flaccid
Spontaneous movements	None	Fasciculations

Reflexes	↑↑	↓↓
Babinski's reflex	Present	Absent
Examples	Stroke, MS	Neuropathy

4. Why is the pain aggravated when he sneezes?

Sneezing increases intra-abdominal as well as intraspinal pressure (Valsalva's maneuver). Neck pain that radiates down the arms in a radicular (nerve root) pattern and that is worsened by a Valsalva's maneuver such as sneezing is highly suggestive of a mass lesion in the cervical spine, such as a herniated cervical disc or tumor. The sneeze causes the mass to exert further pressure on a spinal nerve root (or the spinal cord), resulting in pain that radiates in a radicular pattern.

5. Why is he complaining of urinary urgency?

Urinary urgency (a sense of having to void) is frequently seen with lesions of the central nervous system affecting descending "upper" autonomic neurons that innervate the bladder. These lesions may be located in the frontal lobes, brain stem, or spinal cord and generally cause urinary symptoms only when they are bilateral. The term *spastic bladder* is often used to describe the urinary urgency associated with a lesion affecting the descending "upper" autonomic neurons.

In this patient, urinary urgency is most likely due to the cervical "mass" causing his neck pain and right upper extremity symptoms. This mass is most likely compressing the cervical spinal cord, resulting in a cervical myelopathy (spinal cord problem).

6. What is meant by a truncal sensory level? Why is it important to look for this pattern of sensory loss in this patient?

Truncal sensory level: A dermatomal level on the trunk, below which sensation to all modalities is diminished. Truncal sensory levels are most often caused by a focal spinal cord lesion, most commonly in the thoracic spinal cord.

It is important to look for this pattern of sensory loss in this patient because all of his exam findings suggest the presence of a myelopathy (spinal cord problem).

7. Why are his triceps muscle stretch reflexes hyperactive?

Hyperactive muscle stretch reflexes suggest an UMN lesion. Because the triceps reflex is mediated by the C7-8 nerve roots, hyperactivity of this reflex can only be seen with lesions *above* the C7 level of the spinal cord, which damage the corticospinal tracts that provide upper motor neuron innervation to the anterior horn cells located in the C7 and C8 ventral horns of the spinal cord.

In this patient, the cervical mass that we are postulating as the cause of all of his other symptoms and signs is most likely compressing the corticospinal tracts in the cervical spinal cord. This compression results in hyperactive triceps reflexes.

8. Can a lesion in one neuroanatomic region explain all of the patient's neurological findings in this patient? Account for all motor, sensory, and autonomic symptoms.

A C5-6 mass, such as a disc protrusion, can compress the spinal cord at this level, causing lower-extremity UMN dysfunction and a spastic bladder. In addition, the mass lesion appears to involve the left side more than the right and to cause compression of the exiting C5-6 dorsal and ventral spinal nerve roots.

More rostral lesions, say in the brain stem or cerebral hemispheres, could not account for the dermatomal sensory loss or absent biceps and brachioradialis reflexes. More caudal lesions in the spinal cord would not explain the hyperactive triceps reflexes. A lesion in the left brachial plexus or left limb peripheral nerves would not explain the hyperactive lower limb reflexes, extensor plantar responses, or spastic bladder.

9. Explain in detail how one lesion could produce LMN signs in the upper extremities and UMN signs in the lower extremities?

A cervical spinal cord lesion can simultaneously damage descending corticospinal tract fibers (UMN) destined for thoracic, lumbar, and sacral levels of the spinal cord, and exiting anterior horn cell axons (LMN) en route to the brachial plexus and upper extremity peripheral nerves.

10. Figure 9 shows sagittal and axial cervical MR scans obtained on admission. What is your diagnosis?

The sagittal MR scan *(A)* shows cervical disc herniations at multiple levels, impinging on the spinal cord and causing a myelopathy. The axial MR scan *(B)* shows a laterally displaced disc, which narrows the C6 neural foramen and impinges on the exiting spinal nerve root. The C5-6 herniated disc is causing a myelopathy *below* the level of the lesion and a radiculopathy *at* the level of the lesion.

11. What different forms of treatment are available for this patient, and what would you recommend?

Medical treatment: Partial neck immobilization by placing the patient in a Philadelphia cervical collar; nonsteroidal anti-inflammatory drugs. Some physicians would also suggest a trial of corticosteroids to reduce any inflammation contributing to the compressive effects of the protruding disc.

Neurosurgical treatment: Surgical decompression of the protruding disc material.

Given the extent of neurological damage being produced by the disc, an urgent neurosurgical referral is indicated. Delaying treatment may result in the damage becoming permanent or in the onset of new neurological deficits, including lower extremity paralysis. Prompt treatment (within days) may effect an improvement in some of this patient's symptoms and signs.

The Grounded Jockey

KEY TERMS

peripheral nervous system: The portion of the nervous system outside the central nervous system; the 12 pairs of cranial nerves and 31 pairs of spinal nerves.

straight leg-raising sign: Pain elicited in response to stretching the sciatic nerve by flexing the hip with the knee extended, usually signifying pathologic damage to the L4, L5, S1, or S2 nerve roots.

antalgic gait: A gait in which the patient experiences pain during the stance phase and thus remains on the painful leg for as short a time as possible.

hypesthesia: A lessened sensibility to touch; variant of hypoesthesia.

radicular pain: Pain in a dermatomal distribution, usually signifying pathologic damage to a single nerve root.

sciatica: Severe pain in the leg along the course of the sciatic nerve felt at the back of the thigh and running down the inside of the leg.

myelogram: A radiograph of the spinal cord and associated nerves.

computed tomography (CT) scan: A method for imaging the body that uses computer-assisted analysis of numerous sectional radiographic images of the body.

HISTORY AND EXAMINATION

History of the Present Illness

A 34-year-old, right-handed jockey at the Finger Lakes Raceway presents to your office with back and leg pain. Six days ago, during the 6th race at Saturday's matinee, the patient was thrown from his horse while jockeying for position in the last turn. As he fell on the muddy racetrack, he struck his buttocks with great force. He immediately experienced a sharp, excruciating low back pain that radiated down the posterior aspect of his right leg. Over the following 6 days, he has remained bedridden because of constant pain. Coughing aggravates the pain. Three days ago, he noticed a numbness in the lateral aspect of his right leg and on the dorsum of his right foot. He reports no bladder difficulties. Ibuprofen has helped little. Because the

Saratoga race season begins in 2 weeks, he is desperate for help. He is otherwise healthy.

Past Medical History

Unremarkable

Medications

None

Physical Examination

He is obviously in pain and prefers to stand. BP = 145/80; P = 92/min. Paralumbar muscle spasms are present, more so on the right.

Neurological Examination

Mental status, cranial nerves, and upper extremities are normal. On functional motor testing, he is unable to stand on his right heel. On formal motor testing, he has the following (R/L): hip flexors 5/5, knee flexors 5/5, knee extensors 5/5, extensor hallucis longus 4+/5, plantar flexors 5/5, ankle dorsiflexors 4+/5. Sensory examination reveals diminished light touch and pinprick over the right posterolateral thigh, right lateral leg, and the dorsum on his right foot. His muscle stretch reflexes are as follows: upper extremities: 2/2, lower extremities: knee jerk 2/2, ankle jerk 2/2. Plantar responses are flexor bilaterally. His gait is antalgic, and he has a positive right straight leg-raising sign.

Questions

1. How do the patient's sensory examination findings help differentiate among a lesion of a peripheral nerve, nerve root, spinal cord, or higher sensory centers? Explain your answer.

2. What is the difference between the cutaneous sensory distribution of peripheral nerves and the cutaneous sensory distribution of nerve roots?

3. Why did the patient have difficulty walking on his right heel? What nerve roots, peripheral nerves, and muscles subserve this function?

4. Why does coughing aggravate his pain?

5. Describe the pathway for the lower motor neurons that are involved in causing leg weakness in this patient, starting from their cell bodies in the anterior horn of the spinal cord and ending in the muscles that are weak. Name the nerve roots and peripheral nerves through which these motor fibers travel.

6. Why does the patient have symmetrical knee and ankle muscle stretch reflexes despite his right leg pain, weakness, and numbness?

7. Localize the patient's lesion. How does the straight leg-raising sign help you?

8. What is your diagnosis?

9. A lumbar myelogram and a lumbosacral CT of this patient's lumbar spine are shown in Figure 10. What do these studies show?

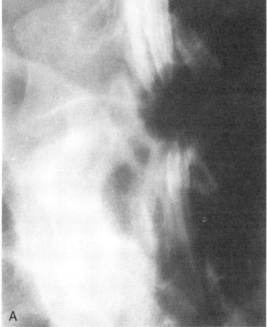

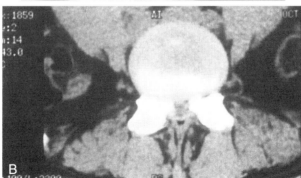

Figure 10. *(A)* Lumbar myelogram. *(B)* Lumbosacral CT scan.

10. How would you manage this patient?

Answers

1. How do the patient's sensory examination findings help differentiate among a lesion of a peripheral nerve, nerve root, spinal cord, or higher sensory centers? Explain your answer.

   The sensory loss seen in this patient (diminished light touch and pinprick over the right posterolateral thigh, right lateral leg, and the dorsum on his right foot) conforms to the sensory distribution of the right L5 nerve root (right L5 dermatome) and is most likely due to a lesion involving this nerve root. A dermatome is a strip of skin supplied by an individual spinal nerve (a nerve root).

   Lesions to peripheral nerves, spinal cord, or more rostral sensory areas produce different patterns of sensory loss. For example, a spinal cord lesion may produce a sensory level below which sensation is impaired. A lesion in the brain stem or more rostral areas may produce a sensory loss on only one side of the body (a hemisensory loss).

2. What is the difference between the cutaneous sensory distribution of peripheral nerves and the cutaneous sensory distribution of nerve roots?

   In lesions of nerve roots, the areas of sensory loss are in the segmental distribution of these nerve roots (dermatomes). In more distal lesions affecting individual peripheral nerves, the areas of sensory loss correspond to the areas of sensory distribution of the specific nerves.

3. Why did the patient have difficulty walking on his right heel? What nerve roots, peripheral nerves, and muscles subserve this function?

   He could not dorsiflex his right foot due to weakness of the tibialis anterior, extensor digitorum longus and brevis, and extensor hallucis longus muscles. Neurons located in the L4 and L5 nerve roots, sciatic nerve, and the deep peroneal nerve innervate these muscles.

4. Why does coughing aggravate his pain?

   He experiences increased intraspinal pressure generated by Valsalva's maneuver during coughing.

5. Describe the pathway for the lower motor neurons that are involved in causing leg weakness in this patient, starting from their cell bodies in the anterior horn of the spinal cord and ending in the muscles that are weak. Name the nerve roots and peripheral nerves through which these motor fibers travel.

   Right L5 nerve root → sciatic nerve → common peroneal nerve → deep peroneal nerve → extensor hallucis longus and tibialis anterior muscles.

6. Why does the patient have symmetrical knee and ankle muscle stretch reflexes despite his right leg pain, weakness, and numbness?

   Because the L5 nerve root does not subserve either muscle stretch reflex.

7 Localize the patient's lesion. How does the straight leg-raising sign help you?

   Right L5 nerve root.

   The straight leg-raising test stretches the sciatic nerve and all of its component nerve roots (L4–S2). A positive straight leg-raising sign suggests L4–S2 nerve root pathology.

8. What is your diagnosis?

   He has a right L5 radiculopathy from a herniated disc.

9. A lumbar myelogram and a lumbosacral CT of this patient's lumbar spine are shown in Figure 10. What do these studies show?

   The lumbar myelogram and the lumbosacral CT show a posterolateral herniated L4-L5 disc with disc material encroaching in on the spinal canal. Although the exact compression of the right L5 nerve root is difficult to discern, the typical disc herniation compresses the nerve root passing to the next intervertebral level. In this case, the L4-L5 disc herniation is compressing the L5 nerve root that exits from the L5-S1 intervertebral foramen.

10. How would you manage this patient?

   Given the presence of objective neurological signs, one would refer the patient for neurosurgery to decompress the herniated disc. While waiting for neurosurgery, one would advise light physical activity and prescribe nonsteroidal anti-inflammatory agents.

The Lumbering Lumberyard Owner

autonomic dysfunction: Dysfunction of one or several components of the autonomic nervous system, the part of the nervous system that controls involuntary bodily functions.

dysarthria: Difficult and defective speech due to impairment of the tongue or other muscles essential to speech. Inability to speak in which there is no defect in the ability to understand and, if literate, to read or write.

aphasia: Absence or impairment of the ability to communicate through speech, writing, or signs because of dysfunction of the dominant brain hemisphere.

dysphagia: Inability to swallow or difficulty in swallowing.

Horner's syndrome: A syndrome characterized by constriction of the pupil, partial ptosis of the eyelid, enophthalmos, and sometimes loss of sweating over one side of the face.

bulbar dysfunction: Dysfunction of muscles innervated by the cranial nerves whose nuclei are found in the medulla; dysphagia and dysarthria.

carotid endarterectomy: A surgical technique for removing intra-arterial obstructions of the lower cervical portion of the internal carotid artery.

HISTORY AND EXAMINATION

History of the Present Illness

An 80-year-old, right-handed, former lumberyard owner comes to your office for a second opinion regarding carotid endarterectomy. One year ago, the patient had three episodes of unsteady gait over a 48-hour period. Each episode lasted about 30 minutes. The patient's wife says that during each of these episodes he looked as if he were going to topple over and that he asked to lie down. There was no headache, double vision, incontinence, or loss of consciousness. On the third morning of these episodes, he awoke unable to walk normally. He required assistance to get to the bathroom, where he complained of dizziness and vomited. His wife noticed that he sounded hoarse. When he attempted to drink coffee, he sputtered, coughed, and spit out the mouthful.

The patient was evaluated at the local hospital, where a computed tomography (CT) scan showed mild generalized atrophy of the brain. Noninvasive carotid testing indicated a 70% stenosis of the right internal carotid artery and a 60% stenosis of the left internal carotid artery. The symptoms improved somewhat over 3 days. After a week of physical therapy, the patient left the hospital against medical advice, saying, "I can do this stuff better at home." He was prescribed warfarin (an oral anticoagulant) for presumed cerebrovascular disease.

During the past year, the patient has experienced difficulty swallowing liquids, choking a number of times. His wife has noticed that his voice remains hoarse. The patient has said that his left side cannot sense temperature any more, causing him to burn his fingers on two occasions. He finds walking difficult at times and often holds onto furniture or onto his wife. He and his wife deny any other neurologic symptoms.

Doctors have urged the patient to have a carotid endarterectomy, and he presents to your office on the advice of his granddaughter, who is a first-year medical student.

Past Medical History

Notable for diabetes mellitus for 5 years, coronary artery disease with a four-vessel coronary artery bypass graft, and emphysema

Medications

Insulin, warfarin, and nitroglycerin

Physical Examination

The patient was obese and in no apparent distress. BP = 124/74 mm Hg; P = 84/min; no postural blood pressure changes. He had bilateral carotid bruits (left greater than right), occasional premature heartbeats but no murmurs, and decreased peripheral pulses.

Neurological Examination

Mental status: Alert, oriented, coherent, no evidence of memory loss, aphasia, or neglect. *Cranial nerves:* Normal except that pupils were (R/L) 2mm/4mm reacting to 1.5/2.5; there was partial ptosis on the right, mild decreased sensation to pain and temperature over the right cheek and chin, dysarthria, dysphagia on drinking water, and a palate that elevated only on the left. *Motor:* Normal strength, tone, and bulk. No tremor. *Sensation:* Decreased to pin and temperature over the left arm, trunk, and leg. *Muscle stretch reflexes:* 2/2 in arms but absent in the legs; plantar responses were flexor bilaterally. *Gait:* Wide-based, with the patient falling to the right on one occasion.

Questions

1. What autonomic nervous system functions are defective in this patient? What is the eponym associated with these dysfunctions? What other autonomic symptoms are associated with this syndrome? Describe in detail the anatomic pathway associated with this syndrome. Is the autonomic dysfunction in this patient the result of a central or peripheral nerve lesion?

2. In a patient with extensive hemisensory loss but no motor abnormalities, where could the lesion be? Where are the pathways for pain and temperature sensation from the left trunk and limbs? For vibration and proprioception sensation from the left trunk and limbs?

3. What is the difference between dysarthria and aphasia? Is this difference significant? Why is this patient hoarse?

4. What does "bulbar musculature" refer to? Which cranial nerves innervate the bulbar musculature? What does "bulb" refer to in this context? What bulbar dysfunction does this patient manifest?

5. Can you explain the patient's crossed sensory findings (right face and left body) with one lesion?

6. Why does this patient have an unsteady gait?

7. Does the patient have more than one lesion? If so, where are they? Can all of the patient's symptoms and signs be localized to one lesion? Where?

8. Is there one blood vessel that can supply all the territory affected in this patient?

9. Is there further testing you would want to do on this patient before making your recommendations to him?

10. If you performed an angiogram, which blood vessel would you expect to find blocked? Should an angiogram be obtained in this patient?

11. Do you agree that this patient should have the carotid endarterectomy?

12. Figure 11 shows a photomicrograph of a pathologic specimen from a patient who died with a similar lesion. Match the neuroanatomic structures that are lesioned on this specimen with this patient's symptoms.

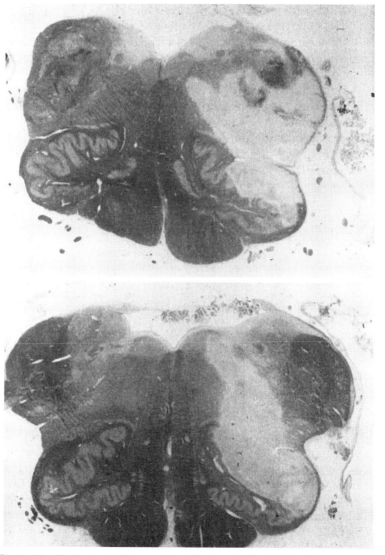

Figure 11. Myelin stain of the medulla at the level of the inferior olives.

Answers

1. What autonomic nervous system functions are defective in this patient? What is the eponym associated with these dysfunctions? What other autonomic symptoms are associated with this syndrome? Describe in detail the anatomic pathway associated with this syndrome. Is the autonomic dysfunction in this patient the result of a central or peripheral nerve lesion?

   The defective autonomic functions are pupillary dilatation and lid elevation.

   The eponym is Horner's syndrome.

   Other symptoms associated with Horner's syndrome include hemianhidrosis (lack of sweating on one half of the face) and enophthalmos ("sunken-in" eyeball).

   Hypothalamus → brain stem reticular formation → cervical spinal cord → synapse on preganglionic sympathetics in the intermediolateral cell column of the spinal cord at T1-T2 → superior cervical ganglion → postganglionic fibers travel with the carotid artery and the first division of the trigeminal nerve to the pupillary dilator muscle (Fig. 12).

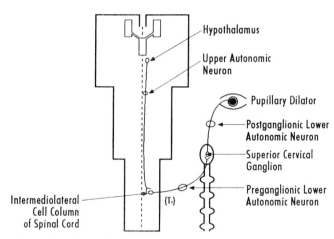

Figure 12. Sympathetic nervous system.

   Considering the other central nervous system (CNS) motor and sensory signs and symptoms such as dysarthia, dysphagia, right facial sensory loss, and left body sensory loss, the lesion causing Horner's syndrome in this patient is most likely located in the CNS (specifically the lateral medulla).

2. In a patient with extensive hemisensory loss but no motor abnormalities, where could the lesion be? Where are the pathways for pain and temperature sensation from the left trunk and limbs? For vibration and proprioception sensation from the left trunk and limbs?

A lesion that produces purely hemisensory symptoms without motor involvement must be located in areas of the CNS where the sensory nuclei and tracts are found separate from motor pathways. Such locations include the lateral spinothalamic tract in the brain stem, the thalamus, or the parietal cortex.

Pain-temperature pathways: Pain and temperature receptors → cross at anterior white commissure (one or two spinal levels up) → anterolateral spinothalamic tract → nucleus ventralis posterolateral (VPL) and nonspecific nuclei of thalamus → primary and secondary sensory cortex (Fig.13).

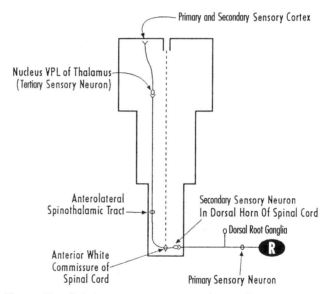

Figure 13. Pain-temperature sensory pathways. R = receptor.

Proprioception-vibration pathways: Encapsulated nerve endings → dorsal columns → nucleus and fasciculus gracilis and cuneatus → cross in the internal arcuate fibers of the medulla and ascend in the medial lemniscus → nucleus VPL of the thalamus → primary and secondary sensory cortex (Fig. 14).

3. What is the difference between dysarthria and aphasia? Is this difference significant? Why is this patient hoarse?

Dysarthria: Motor difficulty with speech implying a brain stem or cerebellar lesion.

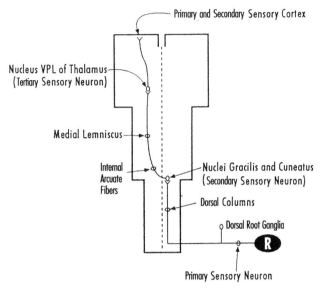

Figure 14. Proprioception-vibration sensory pathways. R = receptor.

Aphasia: An acquired dysfunction of language implying a cortical lesion.

Because all of the patient's other motor, sensory, and autonomic symptoms also localize to the medulla, his hoarseness is most likely due to vocal cord paralysis as a result of damage to the nucleus ambiguus in the lateral medulla.

4. What does "bulbar musculature" refer to? Which cranial nerves innervate the bulbar musculature? What does "bulb" refer to in this context? What bulbar dysfunction does this patient manifest?

The bulbar musculature refers to muscles of the pharynx, larynx, and tongue, which are innervated by cranial nerves IX, X, XI, and XII.

The "bulb" refers to the medulla.

This patient has dysarthria and dysphagia, which are due to dysfunction of the lower cranial nerves and likely due to a lesion in the medulla.

5. Can you explain the patient's crossed sensory findings (right face and left body) with one lesion?

The crossed sensory findings in this patient (right face and left body) are most likely due to a lesion in the right lateral medulla, which affects the descending nucleus and tract of the trigeminal nerve, causing ipsilateral facial numbness (Figs.15 and 16), and the spinothalamic tract, causing contralateral

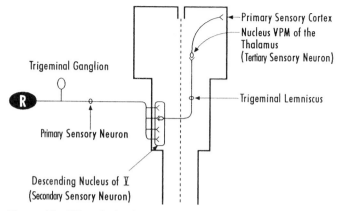

Figure 15. Trigeminal pain-temperature sensory pathways. VPM = ventral posteromedial, R = receptor.

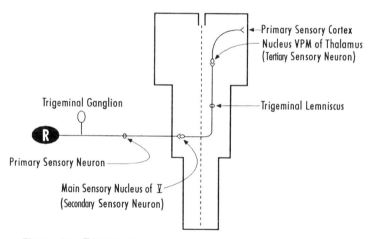

Figure 16. Trigeminal proprioception-vibration sensory pathways. VPM = ventral posteromedial, R = receptor.

body numbness (Fig. 13). No other single location in the CNS can result in these sensory findings.

6. Why does this patient have an unsteady gait?

His unsteady gait is probably caused by a lesion involving the inferior cerebellar peduncle in the lateral medulla. Although unsteady gait has many causes (cerebellar lesions, lesions to peripheral nerves or to the posterior columns, upper motor neuron or basal ganglia lesions), all of his other signs and symptoms localize to the lateral medulla.

7. Does the patient have more than one lesion? If so, where are they? Can all of the patient's symptoms and signs be localized to one lesion? Where?

Most likely the patient has one lesion in the lateral medulla. This lesion explains all of his symptoms and signs, as follows:

Symptom or Sign	Structure Affected in the Lateral Medulla
Unsteady gait	Inferior cerebellar peduncle
Dizziness and vomiting	Vestibular nuclei
Hoarseness	Nucleus ambiguus
Dysphagia	Nucleus ambiguus
Left body numbness	Spinothalamic tract (spinal lemniscus)
Right facial numbness	Descending nucleus and tract of cranial nerve V
Horner's syndrome	Descending sympathetic fibers

This lesion does not explain the loss of lower extremity reflexes, but this loss is explained by the coexistence of a diabetic polyneuropathy.

8. Is there one blood vessel that can supply all the territory affected in this patient?

The posterior inferior cerebellar artery supplies the lateral medulla.

9. Is there further testing you would want to do on this patient before making your recommendations to him?

Further testing in this patient would include an electrocardiogram (ECG) and possible echocardiogram to rule out a cardiac source of emboli. Because this patient has already had one stroke, it is imperative that his risk for further stroke be minimized.

A magnetic resonance (MR) scan of the brain would likely show the lesion in the lateral medulla, but such a scan is probably not necessary because his signs and symptoms are sufficient to localize the stroke with great precision.

10. If you performed an angiogram, which blood vessel would you expect to find blocked? Should an angiogram be obtained in this patient?

The right vertebral artery, which gives rise to the right posterior inferior cerebellar artery, is most likely to be blocked.

There is no need to obtain an angiogram in this patient because findings on angiography would not change his treatment. Arteries in the posterior circulation are too small to lend themselves to surgical recanalization.

11. Do you agree that this patient should have the carotid endarterectomy?

No, because his symptoms are due to an ischemic infarct in the posterior circulation (vertebrobasilar system), not in the anterior circulation (internal carotid system). The stenosis of his carotid arteries found on ultrasonography has not caused any clinical symptoms and is an incidental finding. Surgery for asymptomatic carotid stenosis is only recommended for severe narrowing of the vessels (>70%).

12. Figure 11 shows a photomicrograph of a pathologic specimen from a patient who died with a similar lesion. Match the neuroanatomic structures that are lesioned on this specimen with this patient's symptoms.

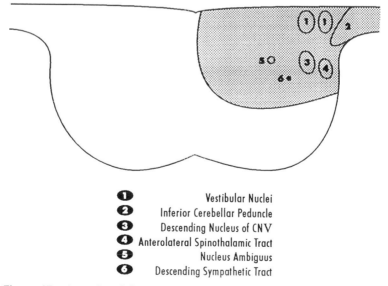

❶	Vestibular Nuclei
❷	Inferior Cerebellar Peduncle
❸	Descending Nucleus of CN V
❹	Anterolateral Spinothalamic Tract
❺	Nucleus Ambiguus
❻	Descending Sympathetic Tract

Figure 17. Lateral medullary syndrome: location of anatomic structures.

Structure	Symptom or Sign
Vestibular nuclei	Dizziness and vomiting
Inferior cerebellar peduncle	Ataxia (unsteady gait)
Descending nucleus of cranial nerve V	Ipsilateral (right) facial numbness
Anterolateral spinothalamic tract	Contralateral (left) body numbness
Nucleus ambiguus	Dysarthria (hoarseness), dysphagia
Descending sympathetic tract	Ipsilateral (right) Horner's syndrome

The Bleary-Eyed Banker

KEY TERMS

diplopia: Double vision.

mitral valve prolapse: A common and occasionally serious condition in which the cusp or cusps of the mitral valve prolapse into the left atrium during systole.

abduction: Lateral movement of a limb or eye away from the median plane of the body.

adduction: Lateral movement of a limb or eye toward the median plane of the body.

direct light reflex: Prompt contraction of the pupillary constrictor muscle of the ipsilateral eye when light entering through the pupil strikes the retina.

consensual light reflex: Prompt contraction of the pupillary constrictor muscle of the contralateral eye when light entering through the pupil strikes the retina.

embolus: A mass of undissolved matter present in a blood vessel and brought there by the blood current.

thrombosis: The formation, development, or existence of a blood clot or thrombus within the vascular system.

homonymous hemianopia: Blindness of nasal half of the visual field of one eye and temporal half of the other, or right-sided or left-sided visual field loss of corresponding sides in both eyes.

HISTORY AND EXAMINATION

History of the Present Illness

A 32-year-old, left-handed woman, who is a loan officer for a local mortgage company, presents to the emergency room with blurry vision. At 9 o'clock this morning, as she was preparing to discuss a mortgage with a 2nd-year medical student and his wife, the patient noticed the sudden onset of painless blurred vision. The cup of coffee she was holding in her right hand slipped out and spilled on the medical student's shirt. "I feel so dizzy," the patient whispered, "I can't see straight."

The alert medical student helped the patient to lie down on the floor. A quick but organized examination revealed that the pulse was faint but regular, the right hand was weaker than the left, and speech was normal. The blurry vision resolved by closing either eye, as did the dizziness. By the time the ambulance arrived, the patient felt much better, but she agreed to go to the emergency room to get things checked out. Slight blurring of vision remained.

Past Medical History

Notable for migraine headaches between 17 and 25 years of age but no previous neurological symptoms. She has a family history of diabetes and gout. A social drinker, she has smoked one pack of cigarettes per day for 13 years.

Medications

Oral contraceptive

Physical Examination

She is anxious. BP = 145/90 mm Hg; P = 96/min; afebrile. Notable for the lack of cervical bruits, symmetrical radial pulses, and a mitral valve prolapse click on cardiac examination.

Neurological Examination

Alert, oriented, and coherent. There is no evidence of memory deficit or aphasia. Visual acuity is 20/15 bilaterally when each eye is tested separately, but 20/100 when tested with both eyes open. Pupils 3 mm/3 mm (R/L) reacting to 2.5/2.5. Visual fields full. Fundi benign. Ocular movements appear conjugate and no nystagmus is seen. The patient prefers to keep one eye closed. When the patient holds a red filter in front of the right eye and looks at a light, the white light always appears lateral to the red light on attempted rightward gaze. All other cranial nerves are normal. A motor examination shows normal strength, tone, and bulk. There is no tremor. Sensation is normal. Muscle stretch reflexes are 1+ and symmetrical. The plantar response is extensor on the right and flexor on the left.

A computed tomography (CT) of the head is normal. Electrocardiogram and blood coagulation studies are normal.

Following the CT scan, the patient notices that she feels much more dizzy. Examination now shows that the left eye does not adduct past the midline or move vertically at all; it does abduct normally. Right eye movements are normal. A right lower facial droop is present and the right arm and leg can barely lift against gravity. Sensation remains normal. Right-sided reflexes are absent and the right plantar response is still extensor. Minutes later, the left pupil enlarges to 6 mm and does not react directly or consensually to light, whereas the right pupil reacts normally.

Questions

1. Why was her vision blurred? How does the "red glass test" help to localize her vision problem?

2. Why were her right-sided reflexes absent? Is this inconsistent with a right-sided plantar extensor response? Why or why not?

3. Where is her lesion? What is the name of the syndrome that produces the combination of signs and symptoms found in this patient?

4. Which blood vessels supply this area? Where do they arise from?

5. What pathologic mechanisms could account for her symptoms?

6. What would happen if a blood clot lodged in the vessel supplying the involved region started extending to surrounding arteries? What other signs might you see? What other symptoms might she experience?

7. Why did the medical student order a head CT scan? What was he looking for?

8. What further tests would you order? How should the patient be treated?

9. What should the patient do in the future to avoid having further such episodes?

Answers

1. Why was her vision blurred? How does the "red glass test" help to localize her vision problem?

   Her vision is blurred because of diplopia.

   The "red glass test" helps in locating the paretic muscle, because the image projected from the paretic eye is farthest from the center when gaze is directed in the direction of action of the paretic muscle. Her test results indicate that the left medial rectus muscle is weak (Fig. 18).

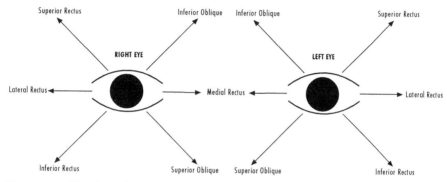

Figure 18. Directions of action of extraocular muscles.

2. Why were her right-sided reflexes absent? Is this inconsistent with a right-sided plantar extensor response? Why or why not?

   An acute upper motor neuron lesion can often produce initial areflexia or hyporeflexia before the onset of hyperreflexia. This is not inconsistent with a plantar extensor response, which indicates an upper motor neuron lesion.

3. Where is her lesion? What is the name of the syndrome that produces the combination of signs and symptoms found in this patient?

   The combination of left cranial nerve III dysfunction and contralateral upper motor neuron dysfunction localizes to the left midbrain.

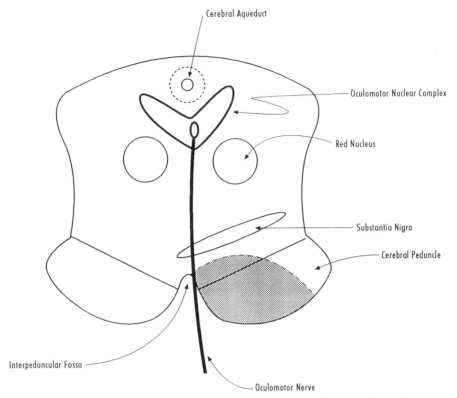

Cerebral Aqueduct

Oculomotor Nuclear Complex

Red Nucleus

Substantia Nigra

Cerebral Peduncle

Interpeduncular Fossa

Oculomotor Nerve

Figure 19. Weber syndrome. The combination of a unilateral oculomotor palsy and contralateral hemiplegia is termed "Weber syndrome." It is due to a lesion (seen as the shaded area in the figure) affecting the dorsal midbrain, involving the cerebral peduncle and exiting fascicles of the oculomotor nerve.

This combination of symptoms is called the Weber syndrome (Fig.19).

4. Which blood vessels supply this area? Where do they arise from?
The vascular supply to the midbrain is from small penetrating arteries arising from the posterior cerebral and basilar arteries.

5. What pathologic mechanisms could account for her symptoms?
Vascular occlusion of the small penetrating arteries subserving the midbrain and resulting in an ischemic infarction (i.e., stroke) could account for her symptoms. Occlusion could result either from thrombotic occlusion of the penetrating arteries or from an embolus arising from a proximal vascular source (e.g., basilar artery, aortic arch, or intracardiac chambers).

6. What would happen if a blood clot lodged in the vessel supplying the involved region started extending to surrounding arteries? What

other signs might you see? What other symptoms might she experience?

If the clot caused impaired blood flow and infarction in the distribution of the left posterior cerebral artery, the patient would also have lack of vision in the right hemifield of both the left and right eyes. This type of blindness is called right homonymous hemianopia. These symptoms could seriously interfere with routine activities such as writing, reading, and driving.

7. Why did the medical student order a head CT scan? What was he looking for?

He ordered a head CT scan to rule out an intracerebral hemorrhage.

8. What further tests would you order? How should the patient be treated?

Further testing: A transesophageal echocardiogram to search for a potential source of cardiac embolus; a head magnetic resonance angiogram to rule out a vertebral artery dissection.

Treatment: Consider antiplatelet agents (aspirin 325 mg/day) or anticoagulants.

9. What should the patient do in the future to avoid having further such episodes?

Beyond medical treatment, she should modify her behavior to reduce the risk of recurrent events. She should be advised to stop smoking and to consider alternative forms of contraception, because oral contraceptive agents may be a risk factor for stroke in young adults (especially with migraine history).

The Silent Secretary

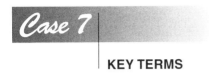

diaschisis: The sudden loss of function in an area that is remote from the causative cerebral lesion but is anatomically connected to it by means of fiber tracts.

hypotonia: Loss of tone of the muscles.

pronator drift: Subtle pronation of the outstretched arm accompanied by abduction and internal rotation at the shoulder and flexion at the elbow, indicative of upper motor neuron dysfunction.

rapid alternating movements: A test of cerebellar hemispheric function performed by asking the patient to alternately slap the thigh with the front and back of the hand or touch each finger to the thumb.

fluent aphasia: Aphasia in which words are easily spoken, but those used are incorrect and may be unrelated to the content of the other words spoken; a sensory, receptive, or Wernicke's aphasia.

nonfluent aphasia: Aphasia in which there is a great difficulty in speaking, although the words produced are usually correct and comprehension of language is unimpaired; a motor, expressive, or Broca's aphasia.

HISTORY AND EXAMINATION

History of the Present Illness

A 60-year-old, right-handed secretary presents to the emergency room with the sudden onset of inability to speak and right hand clumsiness. Her symptoms began abruptly that morning while returning from the bathroom. There was some resolution of her symptoms over the next few hours, but when her daughter called, she noted that her mother's speech was halting and limited. She therefore called an ambulance. Lately, the mother had noted intermittent palpitations but no chest pain, dyspnea, or syncope.

Past Medical History

Two-year history of mild essential hypertension

Medications

Hydrochlorothiazide (a diuretic used to treat hypertension)

Physical Examination

Alert, rubbing the left side of her head; BP = 150/90 mm Hg; P = 110/min; her rhythm is irregularly irregular.

Neurological Examination

She is able to follow simple commands and appears to comprehend conversational speech, but her responses are effortful and limited to simple one-word answers. She is unable to read aloud and can only write her name. On motor examination, her right arm is hypotonic. She has a mild right lower facial droop and right upper extremity weakness. She has a right pronator drift. Her right-hand rapid alternating movements are slowed. Her lower extremities are normal. She has no sensory deficits. There is relative hyporeflexia in the right arm. She has a right plantar extensor response.

Laboratory studies reveal a normal hematocrit and normal electrolytes and glucose. Her electrocardiogram shows atrial fibrillation with a ventricular rate of 90 to 120/min. A head computed tomography (CT) scan obtained that evening is unremarkable.

Within 2 days, her monoparesis has resolved and her speech has become fluent, although she continues to have subtle word-finding difficulties.

Questions

1. How would you characterize the patient's difficulty in communicating? Where does language localize in the brain? What is the difference between fluent and nonfluent aphasia?

2. What is a pronator drift? What does it signify?

3. Why was only her right *lower* face weak?

4. What is the corticobulbar tract? How does it differ from the corticospinal tract?

5. Do you think this patient's weakness is on the basis of upper or lower motor neuron problems? Why? How do you explain her relative hypotonia and hyporeflexia?

6. Localize this patient's lesion.

7. What is this patient's diagnosis? What is the likely pathophysiology? What is the importance of her laboratory data?

8. Why is her CT scan normal? What further diagnostic tests would you recommend?

9. Given her presumed disease mechanism, what treatment would you recommend? What is her prognosis for recovery?

Answers

1. How would you characterize the patient's difficulty in communicating? Where does language localize in the brain? What is the difference between fluent and nonfluent aphasia?

   She has nonfluent expressive aphasia.

   Language localizes to the frontal and parietal lobes of the dominant hemisphere (Fig. 20).

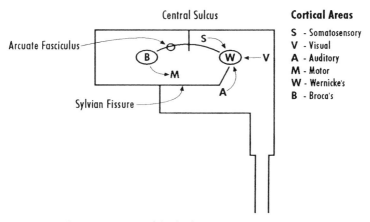

Figure 20. Language areas of the brain.

   Fluent (receptive, sensory, Wernicke's) aphasia: Patient maintains normal rhythm and cadence, but comprehension and word content are impaired.

   Nonfluent (expressive, motor, Broca's) aphasia: Rhythm and cadence are markedly abnormal; comprehension is intact.

2. What is a pronator drift? What does it signify?

   One elicits a pronator drift by having patients hold out their arms in the supinated and extended position. The patients then close their eyes and are distracted by being asked to shake their head side-to-side (saying "no"). A pronator drift is present when an arm pronates, abducts, and internally rotates. This signifies weakness due to an upper motor neuron (UMN) lesion.

3. Why was only her right *lower* face weak?

   The upper face has bilateral UMN (corticobulbar) innervation. Therefore, a unilateral UMN lesion will cause contralateral weakness only to the lower face. The upper face can become weak, with bilateral corticobulbar lesions or with peripheral cranial nerve VII lesions.

4. What is the corticobulbar tract? How does it differ from the cortico-spinal tract?

Corticobulbar tract: UMN innervation to the brain stem motor nuclei (Fig. 21). The tract has both ipsilateral (uncrossed)

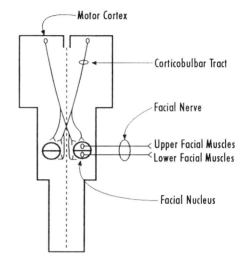

Figure 21. The corticobulbar system to the face.

and contralateral (crossed) innervation to all motor nuclei except the lower face, which has only crossed innervation.

Corticospinal tract: UMN innervation to the spinal cord anterior horn cells (Fig. 22). This tract is mainly crossed (decussation of the pyramids).

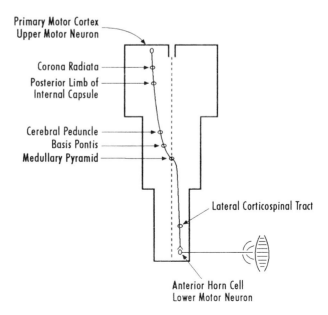

Figure 22. The cortico-spinal system.

5. Do you think this patient's weakness is on the basis of upper or lower motor neuron problems? Why? How do you explain her relative hypotonia and hyporeflexia?

UMN, because of the the right pronator drift, right plantar extensor response, and associated aphasia.

Acute forms of hypotonia and hyporeflexia can be seen in UMN lesions (diaschisis).

6. Localize this patient's lesion.

Left frontal lobe, affecting Broca's area and the lateral motor strip.

7. What is this patient's diagnosis? What is the likely pathophysiology? What is the importance of her laboratory data?

She has an ischemic cerebral infarction. The most likely etiology is embolic occlusion of her middle cerebral artery. Atrial fibrillation is a risk factor for emboli.

8. Why is her CT scan normal? What further diagnostic tests would you recommend?

The area of infarction is relatively small, and the time interval from symptom onset to the CT scan is relatively short (12 hours). It often takes 24 to 48 hours to visualize an ischemic infarction on head CT.

Further testing: Echocardiogram (preferably a transesophageal echocardiogram).

9. Given her presumed disease mechanism, what treatment would you recommend? What is her prognosis for recovery?

Treatment: Long-term anticoagulation therapy with oral warfarin. One must take warfarin for several days before the blood is sufficiently anticoagulated. During this period of waiting, she should be placed on intravenous heparin. Digoxin should also be added to control atrial fibrillation.

Prognosis: Relatively good because emboli frequently disintegrate, and the risk of recurrence is low while therapeutic anticoagulation is administered.

The Comatose Custodian

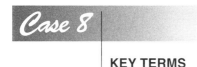

KEY TERMS

hyperpnea: An increased respiratory rate or breathing that is deeper than that usually experienced during normal activity.

apnea: Temporary cessation of breathing.

Cheyne-Stokes respiration: A common and bizarre breathing pattern marked by a period of apnea lasting 10 to 60 seconds, followed by gradually increasing depth and frequency of respiration.

extensor (decerebrate) posturing: A posture exhibiting uninhibited extension of all four extremities and seen with lesions to the midbrain; decerebrate rigidity.

anisocoria: Inequality of the size of the pupils.

intracranial pressure: The pressure of the cerebrospinal fluid in the subarachnoid space between the skull and the brain.

cerebral herniation: A condition in which local pressure gradients from focal brain lesions shift the rather fluid brain substance in relation to the rigid falx, tentorium, or foramen magnum.

uncal herniation: An infrequently seen form of cerebral herniation with large mass lesions in the temporal lobe. The uncus herniates across the free edge of the tentorium, compressing the third cranial nerve and the cerebral peduncle, and producing ipsilateral pupillary dilatation, ptosis and ophthalmoplegia, as well as contralateral spastic hemiparesis, hyperreflexia, and Babinski's sign.

HISTORY AND EXAMINATION

History of the Present Illness

A 55-year-old custodian was found by his family unresponsive in the bathroom, with vomitus on the floor. He was rushed to the emergency department. The family reports that he was a heavy drinker and that the last time he saw a physician (15 years ago), he was told he had hypertension. Over the last 1 to 2 weeks, he had been complaining of headaches, which seemed to lessen in severity following increased alcohol consumption.

Past Medical History

Frequent headaches

Medications

Aspirin, taken on an "as needed" basis for his headaches

Physical Examination

He is lying motionless with his eyes closed. BP = 250/120 mm Hg; P = 100/min, regular; R = 20/min, alternating hyperpnea and apnea.

Neurological Examination

He is unresponsive to verbal or tactile stimuli. With noxious stimulation, he has semipurposeful movements of the right upper extremity, but the left side exhibits extensor posturing. His fundi reveal moderate arteriolar narrowing and arteriovenous nicking but no papilledema. His pupils are anisocoric (R/L = 3.5 mm/2.0 mm), but both react to light, although the right is more sluggish. He has spontaneous roving conjugate eye movements but tends to look to the right. His eyelid tone is diminished on the left, and he has flattening of the left nasolabial fold. His left side is flaccid with external rotation of his left leg. He has bilateral plantar extensor responses.

He was intubated, hyperventilated, and taken to the computed tomography (CT) scanner.

Questions

1. What structures are necessary to maintain consciousness? Which of these are involved in this patient?

2. What does extensor (decerebrate) posturing signify? What is decorticate posturing?

3. What is the term for alternating periods of apnea and hyperpnea? What does this sign indicate?

4. Why does the patient tend to look to the right?

5. Why does this patient have anisocoria (unequal pupils)? List four other causes of anisocoria.

6. The patient's head CT scan is shown in Figure 23. Figure 24 shows a coronal cut of a brain specimen from a patient who died with a similar condition. What is your diagnosis?

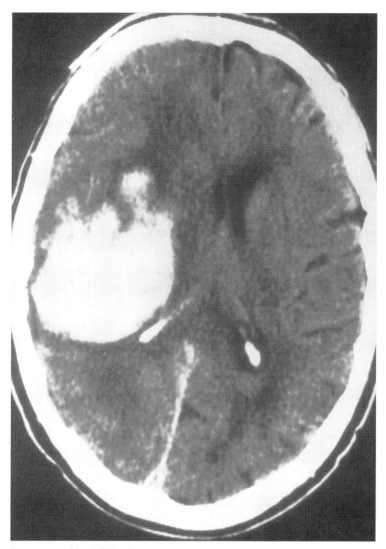

Figure 23. Head CT without contrast.

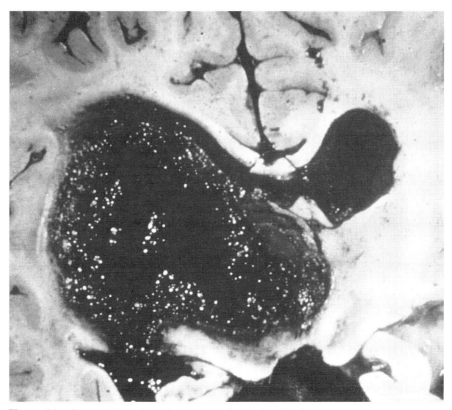

Figure 24. Gross pathologic brain specimen (coronal section).

7. How can his lesion cause coma? Right eye deviation? Left extensor posturing? Cheyne-Stokes respiration? Anisocoria with a large and sluggish right pupil? The diagram in Figure 25 may help you answer this question.

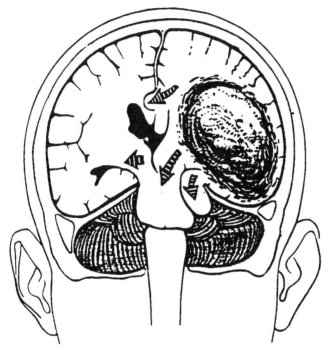

Figure 25. Diagram illustrating mass effect due to an intrahemispheric mass lesion with cingulate, uncal, and transtentorial herniation.

8. What is the cause and location of this patient's lesion? What other locations in the brain are susceptible to this process?

9. Why was the patient intubated and hyperventilated? Would you recommend other treatments or tests at this time?

10. Why might this patient acutely deteriorate in the next several days? What is the prognosis?

11. If this patient survives the acute phases of his illness, what are his long-term deficits likely to be?

Answers

1. What structures are necessary to maintain consciousness? Which of these are involved in this patient?

    The necessary structures are the reticular activating system and at least one cerebral hemisphere. Most likely, this patient has diffuse injury affecting both hemispheres and the reticular activating system in the brain stem, although the right cerebral hemisphere is most severely affected.

2. What does extensor (decerebrate) posturing signify? What is decorticate posturing?

    Decerebrate posturing: Extension of legs and extension and external rotation of arms (Fig. 26). This posturing signifies a lesion below the red nucleus in the midbrain.

    Decorticate posturing: Extension of legs and flexion of arms. This signifies a lesion above the red nucleus, often in the diencephalon.

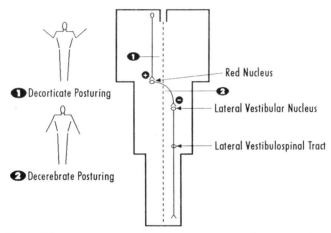

Figure 26.   Motor posturing: decorticate and decerebrate posturing.

3. What is the term for alternating periods of apnea and hyperpnea? What does this sign indicate?

    This is called Cheyne-Stokes respiration. It indicates bihemispheric dysfunction.

4. Why does the patient tend to look to the right?

    He has a destructive lesion in the right hemisphere, ablating the right frontal eye fields. The excitatory action of the left frontal eye fields is unopposed, causing a rightward gaze preference ("looking toward the lesion") (Fig. 27).

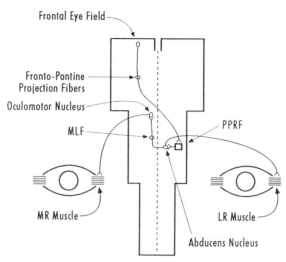

Figure 27. Cortical control of eye movements. LR Muscle = lateral rectus muscle, MR Muscle = medial rectus muscle, MLF = medial longitudinal fasciculus, PPRF = paramedian pontine reticular formation.

5. Why does this patient have anisocoria (unequal pupils)? List four other causes of anisocoria.

The right oculomotor nerve (CN III) is being compressed by uncal herniation, causing a parasympathoparesis. This results in a large, sluggishly reactive right pupil compared to the left.

Other causes of anisocoria are:
• Horner's syndrome
• Adie's syndrome
• Congenital
• Pharmacological

6. The patient's head CT scan is shown on Figure 23. Figure 24 is a coronal cut of a brain specimen from a patient who died with a similar condition. What is your diagnosis?

A large intracerebral hemorrhage: bleeding from an arterial source directly into the brain substance. The noncontrasted head CT scan reveals a massive, right hemispheric acute hemorrhage with prominent mass effect and midline shift. The gross pathologic brain specimen reveals a massive right intracerebral hemorrhage in the region of the basal ganglia, internal capsule, and thalamus, extending into the ventricular system. There is not only a large blood clot but also a marked midline shift.

7. How can his lesion cause coma? Right eye deviation? Left extensor posturing? Cheyne-Stokes respiration? Anisocoria with a large and sluggish right pupil? The diagram shown in Figure 25 may help you answer this question.

Symptom	Cause
Coma	Hemorrhage damaging structures required to maintain consciousness
Right eye deviation	Damage to the frontal eye field
Left extensor posturing	Damage to the right midbrain (below the red nucleus) from compressive effects of the hemorrhage
Cheyne-Stokes respiration	Bihemispheric dysfunction
Anisocoria	Uncal herniation causing a compressive third-nerve paresis

8. What is the cause and location of this patient's lesion? What other locations in the brain are susceptible to this process?

Hypertensive intracerebral hemorrhage into the right basal ganglia.

Other common locations for hypertensive intracerebral hemorrhages include the cerebellum, pons, thalamus, and the gray-white matter junction.

9. Why was the patient intubated and hyperventilated? Would you recommend other treatments or tests at this time?

Patients who are comatose (have a depressed level of consciousness) have a difficult time controlling and clearing their airways from continuous respiratory secretions and are at risk for developing aspiration pneumonias. Endotracheal intubation with artificial respiratory support helps to protect the respiratory airways during periods of depressed consciousness. When coma is caused by increased intracranial pressure, controlled hyperventilation can decrease intracranial pressure. Intracranial pressure can also be decreased with osmotic therapy using mannitol.

10. Why might this patient acutely deteriorate in the next several days? What is the prognosis?

Because increasing cerebral edema can occur over the next 48 to 72 hours. Increasing cerebral edema increases intracranial pressure, which can worsen cerebral herniation with further compression of vital brain stem structures.

Prognosis: Variable. If he survives the next several days, he likely will have severe persistent neurological deficits.

11. If this patient survives the acute phase of his illness, what are his long-term deficits likely to be?

They are likely to be a combination of right hemispheric deficits, including left visual field cut, left hemiplegia, spatial-perceptual difficulties, and left-sided neglect.

The Awkward Dairy Farmer

KEY TERMS

extinction to double simultaneous stimulation: Inability to identify a stimulus on the side of the body contralateral to a parietal lobe lesion, when it is presented simultaneously with a stimulus on the opposite side of the body; sensory neglect.

biceps jerk: A reflex contraction of the biceps brachii, produced by tapping over the insertion of the tendon at the head of the radius.

knee jerk: The extension of the lower leg upon striking the patellar tendon when the knee is flexed at a right angle.

ankle jerk: Contraction of the calf muscles, produced by tapping the stretched Achilles tendon.

ataxia: Defective muscular coordination, especially that manifested when voluntary muscular movements are attempted.

Romberg's test: A functional test of the balance system, in which the patient is observed to see if balance can be maintained with the eyes closed and feet close together. Romberg's test is reported as positive if the patient falls to one side, which implies dysfunction of either the vestibular system or proprioception.

HISTORY AND EXAMINATION

History of the Present Illness

A 72-year-old, right-handed dairy farmer with diabetes mellitus was admitted to the hospital for treatment of a severely infected foot ulcer. On the morning after admission, while eating breakfast, he dropped his coffee cup and spilled coffee on his bed. When the nurse asked him what had happened, he explained that he was not sure but had noticed steady deterioration in his ability to use his right arm since he awoke that morning. The doctor was called. The patient denied any pain or numbness in his right arm or any other neurological symptoms. He also reported no prior similar episodes.

Past Medical History

Notable for coronary artery disease, diabetes mellitus and hypertension

Medications

Lisinopril for hypertension, insulin for diabetes

Physical Examination

He appears well and is lying in bed comfortably. BP = 150/90 mm Hg; P = 100/min. There are no carotid bruits; there is a soft systolic heart murmur that radiates along the left sternal border. Peripheral pulses are diminished.

Neurological Examination

He is alert and has normal language function. The pupils are 5 mm in diameter and react briskly to 3 mm bilaterally. Visual fields are full to confrontation. Ocular motility is full and there is no nystagmus. A mild right facial droop is present. His tongue and palate move normally. On motor examination, he has normal tone with some decrease in distal muscle bulk and strength. On functional testing, he is able to lift his right arm over his head, but a right pronator drift is present. On formal testing, right elbow flexion and extension are weak, and he can barely open his right hand fully. On sensory examination, he has a symmetric decrease, in a distal-to-proximal gradient, of pin, touch, temperature, and vibration. However, he does not extinguish to double simultaneous stimulation. The right biceps and knee jerks are brisker than the left, and no ankle jerks can be obtained. He has a right plantar extensor response. These reflex asymmetries were not present on admission. Gait cannot be tested because of his foot ulcer.

Questions

1. Is his right side weak because of upper motor neuron or lower motor neuron problems? Why?

2. Are his symmetric distal sensory loss and absent ankle jerk reflexes due to disease in the central or peripheral nervous system? Why?

3. Are there any signs of brain stem dysfunction? Cortical dysfunction?

4. Where would you localize the lesion causing his right-sided weakness? Be as specific as possible. Does the absence of focal sensory findings help?

5. What is the etiology of this man's right-sided weaknesses? His distal sensory loss? His diminished muscle bulk? What risk factors does
he possess that predispose him to these findings?

6. Would you expect this patient to be ataxic with his right arm? With his left arm?

7. What would you expect his gait to be? What would Romberg's testing reveal?

8. What further testing would be helpful? What treatment would you recommend? What is his long-term prognosis?

9. What is a lacunar stroke? What are the four most common locations for lacunar strokes?

10. Figures 28 and 29 show two examples of lacunar infarcts that can cause symptoms similar to those that this patient experienced. Describe in detail the location of the infarcts on these images.

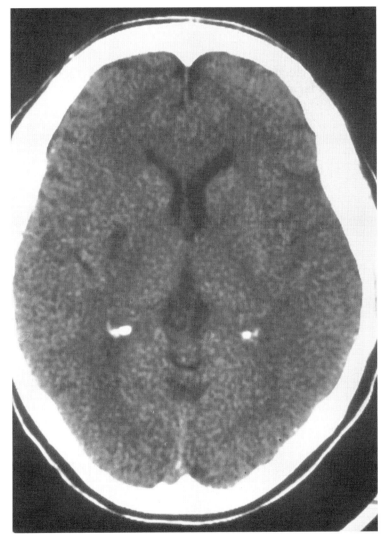

Figure 28.   Head CT scan, without contrast. Patient's right side is on left side of the image and vice versa.

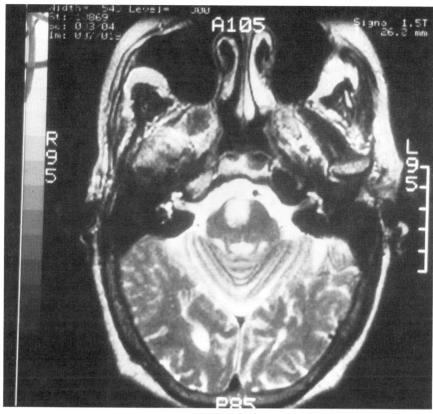

Figure 29. T2-weighted head MR scan. Note "R" and "L."

Answers

1. Is his right side weak because of upper motor neuron or lower motor neuron problems? Why?

   It is weak because of upper motor neuron problems, considering the pronator drift, right-sided hyperreflexia, and right plantar extensor response. Lower motor neuron weakness causes muscle atrophy and hyporeflexia.

2. Are his symmetric distal sensory loss and absent ankle jerk reflexes due to disease in the central or peripheral nervous system? Why?

   They are due to disease in the peripheral nervous system, because areflexia is commonly seen with lower motor neuron problems, and a symmetric distal sensory loss is a pattern commonly seen with peripheral neuropathies ("stocking-glove" or "dying-back" neuropathies). Central nervous system dysfunction often causes hemisensory loss and hyperreflexia.

3. Are there any signs of brain stem dysfunction? Cortical dysfunction?

   Neither. Brain stem signs include the four d's: diplopia, dysphagia, dysarthria, and dysmetria, none of which the patient has. Cortical signs include the four a's: aphasia, apraxia, agnosia, and anopsia. He has none of these either.

4. Where would you localize the lesion causing his right-sided weakness? Be as specific as possible. Does the absence of focal sensory findings help?

   Left internal capsule or basis pontis.

   A lesion to any of these areas can produce "pure motor findings" without sensory abnormalities.

5. What is the etiology of this man's right-sided weaknesses? Of his distal sensory loss? Of his diminished muscle bulk? What are the risk factors that predispose him to these findings?

   His acute right-sided weakness represents a lacunar (small-vessel thrombotic) infarct, most likely due to his history of diabetes mellitus and hypertension.

   His distal sensory loss and diminished muscle bulk are consistent with peripheral neuropathy, most likely due to diabetes mellitus.

6. Would you expect this patient to be ataxic with his right arm? With his left arm?

   He would probably have some slight ataxia with his right arm because of upper motor neuron weakness. One would not expect left-arm ataxia in this patient.

7. What would you expect his gait to be? What would Romberg's testing reveal?

     Most likely, he would have a mixed gait disorder: wide-based caused by peripheral neuropathy and hemiparetic caused by the stroke.

     Romberg's test would be positive due to the peripheral neuropathy.

8. What further testing would be helpful? What treatment would you recommend? What is his long-term prognosis?

     Further testing: Computed tomography (CT) of the head to rule out a hemorrhagic stroke, carotid doppler studies, and possibly a transesophageal echocardiogram.

     Treatment: Risk factor modification—treating the hypertension and diabetes. He should also be started on an antiplatelet agent.

     Prognosis: He is at increased risk of having subsequent strokes.

9. What is a lacunar stroke? What are the four most common locations for lacunar strokes?

     A lacunar stroke is a small brain infarct caused by occlusion of small, deep, penetrating arterioles.

     The four most common locations for lacunar strokes are the internal capsule, pons, thalamus, and basal ganglia.

10. Figures 28 and 29 show two examples of lacunar infarcts that can cause symptoms similar to those that this patient experienced. Describe in detail the location of the infarcts on these images.

     The noncontrasted head CT scan in Figure 28 reveals a small, well-circumscribed hypodense (dark) ischemic infarction in the right putamen extending into the right internal capsule. Note the calcified choroid plexus in the posterior horns of the lateral ventricles.

     The head magnetic resonance scan in Figure 29 reveals a high-signal (bright) lesion in the left basis pontis, representing an ischemic pontine infarction.

The Feeble Gardener

KEY TERMS

gag reflex: Gagging resulting from irritation of the throat or pharynx.

fasciculation: Spontaneous contraction of all of the muscle fibers belonging to a single motor unit that does not cause movement at a joint.

fibrillation: Spontaneous contraction of an individual muscle fiber.

bulbar palsy: Palsy caused by degeneration of the nuclei of the lower cranial nerves.

pseudobulbar palsy: Palsy caused by degeneration of the nuclei of the corticobulbar tracts bilaterally.

electromyography (EMG): The recording and study of spontaneous and voluntary electrical activity of muscle.

HISTORY AND EXAMINATION

History of the Present Illness

E.F., a 70-year-old, right-handed man, sees his physician because of progressive difficulty walking for the past year.

The patient first noted weakness in his legs about a year ago and reports that he has had to use the banister to go upstairs over the past 6 months. Also, in order to stand from sitting, he now has to push down on the arms of the chair. He also complains that when working in the garden he has trouble holding up his head when stooping over and weeding. Typically, after a busy morning in the garden, he has difficulty holding his head up to eat lunch or read the newspaper.

In addition, over the past few months he has noticed that if he drinks too quickly he might cough and choke. Over the past few weeks, the choking has become more serious. On one occasion, his wife had to perform a Heimlich maneuver because he was choking on a pork chop. E.F. adds that his choking does not bother him as much as the fact that he does not feel that he can cough hard enough to clear his airway. Finally, E.F. says that he has stopped talking to friends on the telephone because his friends complain that it is difficult to understand him.

Past Medical History

Significant for coronary artery disease; his only medication is one aspirin daily.

Medications

Aspirin for prevention of vascular disease

Physical Examination

E.F. looks thin and wasted in his face and arms, despite his big torso. BP = 160/86 mm Hg; P = 72/min; R = 14/min, unlabored. Although his lungs are clear, the breath sounds are diminished, and he has a very weak cough. His heart and abdomen are unremarkable, and there are no carotid bruits.

Neurological Examination

His mental status is intact. On cranial nerve examination, he has full visual fields and symmetrically reactive pupils. His fundi are normal, and his ocular movements are full. His face is symmetrically strong, but he has difficulty holding his mouth open against resistance. He is unable to clearly enunciate repeatedly, "Coca-Cola, Coca-Cola." His tongue has normal bulk and strength, but it is difficult for him to protrude it. Although his palate hardly moves when he says "Ah," his gag reflex is very brisk. On motor testing, he is spastic in his upper and lower extremities. Functionally, he cannot lift his head off the bed when lying flat on his back, and he cannot lift his arms above his head. However, he is able to walk on his heels and toes. Formal power is as follows (R/L): Neck flexors 2, biceps 4/4, wrist extensors 5−/5−, finger flexors 4/4, hip flexors 4−/4, knee extensors 4/4+ (no extension lag). Twitching is seen under the skin in his triceps and hand muscles as well as in both anterior tibial compartments. His sensory and cerebellar examinations are normal. His reflexes are very brisk in the upper extremities and he has clonus at the knees and ankles bilaterally. Plantar responses are extensor bilaterally. He walks with stiff legs and a stooped posture, his chin almost resting on his chest.

Questions

1. Is this patient's weakness due to lower motor neuron (LMN) disease? To upper motor neuron (UMN) disease? To both?

2. Both spasticity and rigidity are forms of increased muscular tone. Define each and give examples of diseases in which each is found. Why is this patient spastic?

3. What is clonus, and what is its significance?

4. Why is this patient having difficulty with speech and swallowing?

5. How can E.F.'s tongue have normal muscle power yet have difficulty protruding?

6. What is bulbar palsy? Pseudobulbar palsy? Is either of these present in this patient?

7. Why is E.F. having difficulty with ambulation?

8. Why is his cough weak?

9. What are fasciculations? How do they differ from fibrillations? Are fasciculations always an abnormal finding?

10. What is the most likely diagnosis for E.F.? What is the prognosis?

11. What do you think EMG sampling of his muscles would reveal?

12. In this disease, which two groups of skeletal muscles are almost never involved?

13. Figures 30 and 31 are photomicrographs of a cross section of the spinal cord (Fig. 30) and the ventral (anterior) horn (Fig. 31) from a patient who died from this condition. What areas of the spinal cord demonstrate neuronal degeneration?

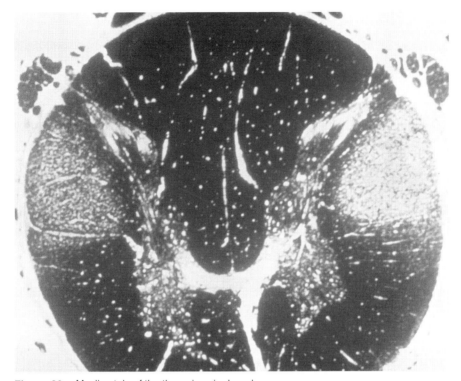

Figure 30.   Myelin stain of the thoracic spinal cord.

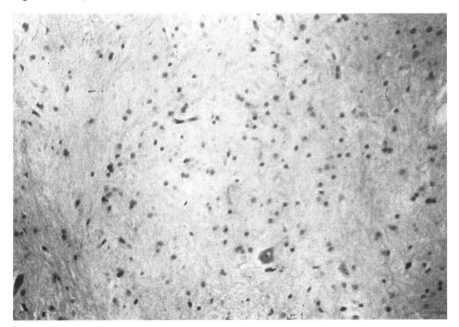

Figure 31.   Hemotoxylin and eosin (H&E) stain from the anterior horn of the spinal cord.

14. Figure 32 shows a normal specimen of skeletal muscle. Figure 33 shows a pathologic specimen of muscle from a patient who died from this condition. What does this muscle specimen show?

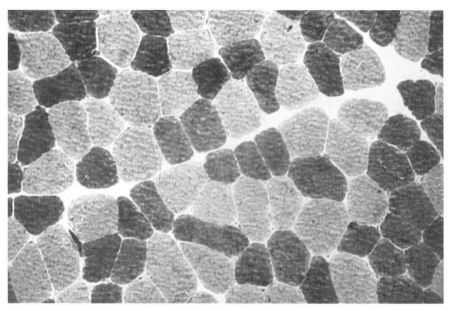

Figure 32. Normal skeletal muscle, routine adenosine triphosphatase (ATPase) stain. In this stain, type 1 muscle fibers stain lightly and type 2 fibers stain darkly. Note the more or less equal numbers of type 1 and type 2 fibers, and the random distribution of these fibers that produces a "mosaic checkerboard" pattern.

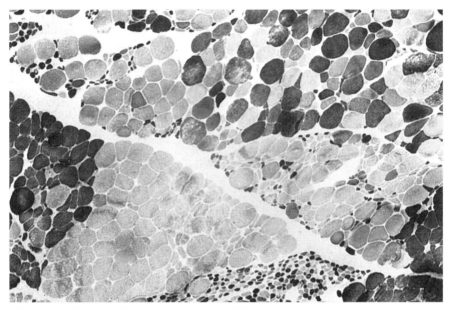

Figure 33. Abnormal skeletal muscle, routine ATPase stain.

15. A gene mutation has been linked to a subset of individuals with the familial form of this condition. What is the enzyme produced by this gene, and on what chromosome is this gene found?

Answers

1. Is this patient's weakness due to lower motor neuron (LMN) disease? To upper motor neuron (UMN) disease? To both?

   To both.

   LMN signs: Muscle wasting, muscle twitching (fasciculations).

   UMN signs: Spasticity, hyperreflexia, Babinski's sign.

2. Both spasticity and rigidity are forms of increased muscular tone. Define each and give examples of diseases in which each is found. Why is this patient spastic?

   Spasticity: Transient, velocity-dependent resistance to passive stretch of muscle, followed by relaxation of the muscle, which results in a "clasp knife" phenomenon. Spasticity may be seen with UMN lesions such as stroke, multiple sclerosis, and motor neuron disease.

   Rigidity: Constant resistance to passive stretch of muscle that is independent of the velocity of movement of the limb, resulting in a "lead pipe" phenomenon. Rigidity may be seen in patients with Parkinson's disease and in patients with other forms of parkinsonism.

   This patient is spastic because his disease process affects the upper motor neurons.

3. What is clonus, and what is its significance?

   Clonus is a repetitive reflex contraction of muscle, frequently elicited in the ankles of patients with extreme hyperreflexia when testing the ankle jerk reflex. Clonus is an upper motor neuron finding and suggests extreme hyperreflexia.

4. Why is this patient having difficulty with speech and swallowing?

   This patient has diffuse muscle weakness that is due to both UMN and LMN dysfunction, as noted above. His difficulty with speech and swallowing most likely represents weakness of the pharyngeal, laryngeal, and tongue muscles. These muscles are known as "bulbar musculature" because they are innervated by lower motor neurons arising from the medulla (the "bulb" of the brain stem). This weakness may be due to either LMN or UMN dysfunction. In this patient, the bulbar weakness is probably UMN in origin, because his tongue has normal bulk (no evidence for atrophy), and his gag reflex is brisk.

5. How can E.F.'s tongue have normal muscle power yet have difficulty protruding?

   Most likely, he has a UMN lesion that affects cortical control of tongue movements. A LMN lesion affecting the hypoglossal nucleus or nerve should produce tongue atrophy, which he does not have.

6. What is bulbar palsy? Pseudobulbar palsy? Is either of these present in this patient?

Bulbar palsy: Weakness and atrophy of the pharynx, larynx, and tongue musculature ("bulbar" musculature) caused by a LMN lesion.

Pseudobulbar palsy: Dysfunction of pharynx, larynx, and tongue musculature caused by bilateral UMN lesions involving the corticobulbar tracts or primary motor cortex. The jaw jerk and gag reflexes are typically brisk in these patients. The term *pseudobulbar* implies that although the bulbar musculature may be weak, there is no lesion to the bulb (medulla) per se but rather to the UMN innervation to the bulb (the pyramidal cells in the primary motor cortex bilaterally, or both corticobulbar tracts).

Recall that, in general, UMN innervation to the brain stem LMNs is *bilateral,* arising from motor cortex in both right and left hemispheres. The only exception to this rule is innervation to the *lower half* of the face, which arises from *contralateral* motor cortex only. For this reason, pseudobulbar palsy only occurs in patients who have sustained bilateral UMN lesions.

Most patients with pseudobulbar palsy also have difficulty controlling their emotions (emotional incontinence) and cry and laugh at inappropriate times. This finding is thought to be a result of an associated degeneration of limbic frontal cortex.

This patient clearly has pseudobulbar palsy, considering the dysarthria and dysphagia, tongue and palate weakness, and the brisk gag reflex.

7. Why is E.F. having difficulty with ambulation?

He has proximal lower extremity weakness and spasticity.

8. Why is his cough weak?

He has chest wall weakness and pharyngeal and laryngeal dysfunction.

9. What are fasciculations? How do they differ from fibrillations? Are fasciculations always an abnormal finding?

Fasciculations: Repetitive firing of individual *motor units,* producing spontaneous contraction but not movement at a joint. Fasciculations are not always abnormal and may be seen with fatigue. Fasciculations can often be seen as "twitching" under the skin.

Fibrillations: Repetitive firing of individual *muscle fibers.*

10. What is the most likely diagnosis for E.F.? What is the prognosis?

   The most likely diagnosis is amyotrophic lateral sclerosis (ALS), also known as Lou Gehrig's disease.

   The prognosis is poor; most patients with ALS die from respiratory failure within 3 years of diagnosis.

11. What do you think EMG sampling of his muscles would reveal?

   Fasciculations and fibrillations, indicating acute denervation caused by death of anterior horn cells and lower motor neurons; large motor units and reduced recruitment of additional motor units with maximal effort, indicating reinnervation of previously denervated motor units and loss of total number of motor units—both signs of chronic denervation.

12. In this disease, which two groups of skeletal muscles are almost never involved?

   Extraocular muscles, and the urinary and bowel sphincter muscles.

13. Figures 30 and 31 are photomicrographs of a cross section of the spinal cord (Fig. 30) and the ventral (anterior) horn (Fig. 31) from a patient who died from this condition. What areas of the spinal cord demonstrate neuronal degeneration?

   The lateral corticospinal tracts (Fig. 30) and anterior horn cells (Fig. 31).

   Figure 30 is a myelin stain of the thoracic spinal cord that reveals myelin loss (resulting from neuronal degeneration) of the lateral columns of the spinal cord in the area of the descending corticospinal tracts.

   Figure 31 is an H&E stain from the anterior horn of the spinal cord that shows one large motor neuron in the lower central portion of the figure. The remaining nerve cells have been destroyed.

14. Figure 32 shows a normal specimen of skeletal muscle. Figure 33 shows a pathologic specimen of muscle from a patient who died from this condition. What does this muscle specimen show?

   Figure 33 shows loss of the normal "mosaic checkerboard" pattern, which results in large groups of type 1 and type 2 muscle fibers. This is known as fiber type grouping and indicates chronic denervation. In this situation, denervated muscle fibers are reinnervated by adjacent axon collateral sprouts, which all belong to a single motor unit; consequently, they will be of the same muscle fiber type. Type grouping and grouped atrophy (not present on this slide) are both seen in muscle biopsy specimens from patients with amyotrophic lateral sclerosis.

15. A gene mutation has been linked to a subset of individuals with the familial form of this condition. What is the enzyme produced by this gene, and on what chromosome is this gene found?

Superoxide dismutase.

On chromosome 21.

The Weak
School Custodian

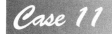
KEY TERMS

diaphoresis: Profuse sweating.

pin sensation: The sensation of sharp pain produced when the skin is touched with the point of a pin.

flaccidity: Defective or absent muscular tone.

cerebrospinal fluid (CSF) examination: An analysis of the cellular, chemical, and microbiologic composition of CSF.

nerve conduction study: A test of the electrophysiologic properties of peripheral nerves, in which a nerve is stimulated electrically, and the amplitude of the evoked potential and the conduction velocity of the nerve are recorded. Nerve conduction studies are useful in evaluating patients with peripheral neuropathies.

plasmapheresis: A procedure in which blood is removed from the body, cellular components are evacuated by use of an automatic blood cell separator device, and plasma is returned to the body by infusion.

HISTORY AND EXAMINATION

History of the Present Illness

S.F., a 26-year-old man, presents to the emergency room because of progressive limb weakness and numbness over the past 2 weeks.

S.F. first noted numbness on both palms 11 days before admission. He described both hands as feeling swollen and prickly. Two days later, he developed the same sort of numbness under his toes. On the following day, he had difficulty climbing stairs or rising from a chair. He denied any other weakness, although he did admit that his wife had to wash his hair for 5 days before coming to the hospital because he could not keep his arms over his head for any length of time. He denied bladder problems but complained of constipation over the past week. He also complained of numbness inside his mouth and that foods tasted salty.

Past Medical History

He has been healthy his whole life but did have a bout of diarrhea 1 month previously. He does not smoke or drink. He works as a school custodian and is a volunteer fireman.

Medications

None

Physical Examination

S.F. appears ill and is profusely diaphoretic. His hands and feet are cool to touch. BP = 140/110 mm Hg; P = 116/min; R = 18/min. His lungs are clear, and his lower back is tender to percussion. He is tachycardic, but cardiac examination is otherwise normal.

Neurological Examination

His mental status is normal. His cranial nerves are also normal except for his inability to bury his eyelashes fully when closing his eyes. He is unable to rise from a chair without pushing with his arms. He is unable to stand on his toes, but he can get up on his heels. His hand grips are weak bilaterally and he cannot make a tight fist. On sensory testing, he has decreased touch, temperature, and vibratory perception below his knees and markedly decreased proprioception at the toes bilaterally. He has normal pin sensation except on the palms of his hands up to the level of the wrists. There is no truncal sensory level. His reflexes are 1+ in the upper extremities, and he has no knee jerk elicitable on the right and only a slight response on the left. No ankle jerks are present, and both plantar responses are flexor.

His admission blood work shows normal blood count and blood chemistries. A CSF examination showed these results:

	S.F.	Normal
WBC	$1/mm^3$	0–5
RBC	$0/mm^3$	0
Glucose	67 mg/dL	>40
Protein	88 mg/dL	25–45

Questions

1. Are this patient's symptoms and signs localized to the central nervous system or the peripheral nervous system?

2. What would you expect his muscle tone to be?

3. Why are his muscle stretch reflexes diminished?

4. Why was this man constipated, diaphoretic, and tachycardic?

5. What is the significance of the CSF findings involving this patient?

6. What is the most likely diagnosis? What is the prognosis? Is any treatment helpful in this disorder?

7. What might you expect nerve conduction studies to show?

8. How might the history of diarrhea be important?

9. How is this disorder different from multiple sclerosis?

Answers

1. Are this patient's symptoms and signs localized to the central nervous system or the peripheral nervous system?

    They are localized to the peripheral nervous system. He has lower motor neuron (LMN) signs (hyporeflexia and absence of Babinski's sign) as well as distal sensory loss in a "stocking-glove" distribution. Both of these findings are most consistent with a peripheral neuropathy (disorder of peripheral nerves).

2. What would you expect his muscle tone to be?

    Decreased (flaccid), because this type of muscle tone is expected in a patient with LMN dysfunction due to a peripheral neuropathy.

3. Why are his muscle stretch reflexes diminished?

    Hyporeflexia (diminished reflexes) is seen with peripheral neuropathies and reflects dysfunction of either the Ia afferent fibers of the monosynaptic stretch reflex (the afferent loop of this reflex) or of the α motor neurons (the efferent loop).

4. Why was this man constipated, diaphoretic, and tachycardic?

    These are all signs of autonomic dysfunction, presumably due to involvement of the peripheral autonomic nerve fibers.

5. What is the significance of the CSF findings involving this patient?

    An elevated CSF protein concentration in the absence of white cells (albumino-cytologic dissociation) is suggestive of a demyelinating polyneuropathy. Myelin is a lipoprotein and in a demyelinating polyneuropathy, breakdown of the myelin coating proximal nerve roots releases protein into the CSF.

6. What is the most likely diagnosis? What is the prognosis? Is any treatment helpful in this disorder?

    Diagnosis: Guillain-Barré syndrome (acute inflammatory demyelinating polyneuropathy).

    Prognosis: Good. Most patients recover within weeks to months, but 35% may have residual deficits.

    Treatments: Plasmapheresis or intravenous immunoglobulin (IVIg), close medical support (including endotracheal intubation and artificial ventilation if necessary), and cardiac monitoring.

7. What might you expect nerve conduction studies to show?

    In most patients with Guillain-Barré syndrome, nerve conduction studies demonstrate prolonged distal sensory and motor latencies and diffusely slowed nerve conduction velocities. These findings are due to the severe demyelination of peripheral nerves, which slows conduction of action potentials in all peripheral nerves. In some patients with mild disease, the result of the nerve conduction study may be normal in the early course of the disease.

8. How might the history of diarrhea be important?

A diarrheal illness suggests an antecedent bacterial (*Campylobacter*) or viral gastroenteritis, which precedes the Guillain-Barré syndrome in about half of the patients.

9. How is this disorder different from multiple sclerosis?

Guillain-Barré syndrome is an *acute*, monophasic illness and is due to *peripheral nervous system* demyelination.

Multiple sclerosis is a *chronic* disease with exacerbations and remissions and is due to *central nervous system* demyelination.

The Tremulous Dentist

KEY TERMS

essential tremor: A tremor, usually involving the head, outstretched hands, and occasionally the voice.

resting tremor: A tremor present when the involved part is at rest but absent or diminished when active movements are attempted.

β-blocker: A substance that blocks the β-adrenergic receptors of the sympathetic nervous system.

mood: A pervasive and sustained emotion that may have a major influence on a person's perception of the world.

affect: The emotional reaction associated with an experience.

cogwheel rigidity: A form of increased muscle tone, typically found at the wrist joint, seen when a resting tremor is superimposed on "lead-pipe" rigidity.

festinating gait: A narrow-based, shuffling gait, in which patients try to catch up with their center of gravity.

HISTORY AND EXAMINATION

History of the Present Illness

J.R. is a 58-year-old, right-handed dentist who is self-referred for the diagnosis of "essential tremor."

J.R. first noted a coarse tremor in his right upper extremity at age 55. Initially, it did not interfere with his technical ability, but over the past year he has had to refrain from more complicated procedures. He was diagnosed with hypertension 2 years ago and after having been placed on a β-blocker, he noted some temporary improvement in this tremor. When specifically questioned, he does acknowledge that he "pushes himself harder" to keep up with his daily schedule. His wife volunteered that he seems less "energetic" and moves more slowly. She thought he was depressed because his facial expression had become less animated.

Past Medical History

He has no other medical problems. There is no history of illicit or psychotropic drug use, head trauma, or exposure to toxins. There is no family history of tremor.

Medications

β-blocker and a thiazide diuretic for hypertension

Physical Examination

J.R. is a meticulously dressed and groomed man. His appearance corresponds to his stated age. His general examination is notable for dry, flaking skin around his eyebrows and hairline. His face is otherwise oily.

Neurological Examination

He has no cognitive, language, or memory deficits. His mood is full, but his affect is blunted. He has a coarse tremor that is most prominent in his hands. The tremor is more pronounced in his right hand and although it is primarily present at rest, it is also present with action. In addition, he has some quivering of his chin but no head tremor. He has "cogwheel" rigidity and diminished finger taps, which are worse on the right. His muscle power and bulk are normal, as is his sensory examination. Cerebellar function is normal. Reflexes are 2+ and symmetrical, and his plantar responses are flexor bilaterally. He has difficulty initiating his gait, and once started, he tends to have difficulty stopping. His steps are small and shuffling and his arm swing is decreased. He also has mild postural instability.

Questions

1. List all of the abnormalities in movement demonstrated by this patient. Is there a name for this syndrome?

2. What is cogwheel rigidity? How does it differ clinically from "lead-pipe" rigidity and from "clasp-knife" spasticity? In which disorders are these abnormalities in tone seen?

3. What is a festinating gait? List another cause for a narrow-based gait with small steps.

4. What is a tremor? Does this patient have "essential tremor"?

5. What is the diagnosis for this patient?

6. What is the pathopharmacology for this man's disease?

7. Figure 34 compares the midbrain of a normal individual with that of one who died from this disease. What is the difference between these two brain specimens?

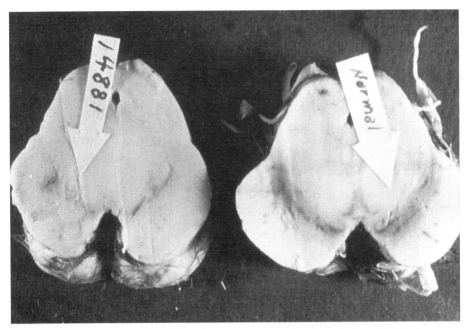

Figure 34. The right side of the figure is a transverse section through the midbrain of a normal individual. At left is a comparable section from a person who died of this man's disease.

8. What are the conventional means of treating this disease? What experimental treatments are currently being tried?

9. Is cognitive decline part of this disease process?

10. What are secondary causes of parkinsonism?

Answers

1. List all of the abnormalities in movement demonstrated by this patient. Is there a name for this syndrome?

    Demonstrated abnormalities include resting tremor, bradykinesia, rigidity, and postural disturbance.

    This syndrome is called parkinsonism.

2. What is cogwheel rigidity? How does it differ clinically from "lead-pipe" rigidity and from "clasp-knife" spasticity? In which disorders are these abnormalities in tone seen?

    Cogwheel rigidity: A resting tremor superimposed on "lead-pipe" rigidity.

    "Lead-pipe" rigidity: A form of increased muscle tone in which there is a constant resistance to passive stretch of a muscle throughout its range of motion. Rigidity is typically seen with all forms of parkinsonism.

    "Clasp-knife" spasticity: Another form of increased muscle tone in which resistance to passive stretch of a muscle *varies with the velocity of stretch*. Spasticity is seen with various upper motor neuron (UMN) disorders such as stroke, multiple sclerosis, and amyotrophic lateral sclerosis.

3. What is a festinating gait? List another cause for a narrow-based gait with small steps.

    Festinating gait: A narrow-based, shuffling gait, in which patients try to catch up with their center of gravity.

    A spastic (scissor) gait is another narrow-based gait, which may be seen with bilateral UMN lesions.

4. What is a tremor? Does this patient have "essential tremor"?

    Tremor: Rhythmic oscillating movements resulting from alternating contractions of opposing muscle groups or from simultaneous contraction of agonist and antagonist muscles.

    This patient does not have *essential* tremor, because essential tremor is an *action* tremor. This patient's tremor is primarily a *resting* tremor.

5. What is the diagnosis for this patient?

    The diagnosis is Parkinson's disease.

6. What is the pathopharmacology for this man's disease?

    Loss of dopamine-containing neurons in the substantia nigra.

7. Figure 34 compares the midbrain of a normal individual with that of one who died from this disease. What is the difference between these two brain specimens?

   The midbrain from the patient who died of Parkinson's disease demonstrates depigmentation of the substantia nigra.

8. What are the conventional means of treating this disease? What experimental treatments are currently being tried?

   Conventional therapy: Anticholinergics, dopamine replacement (carbidopa/levodopa), dopamine agonists (bromocriptine or pergolide), selegiline, and amantadine.

   Experimental therapies: Transplantation of fetal or adrenal medullary cells to the caudate nucleus; pallidotomies; thalamotomies.

9. Is cognitive decline part of this disease process?

   Yes, in some patients, particularly in advanced stages of the disease.

10. What are secondary causes of parkinsonism?

    Drug-induced: Phenothiazines, haloperidol, methyl-phenyl-tetrahydropyridine (MPTP).

    Degenerative: Striato-nigral degeneration, progressive supranuclear palsy, multisystem atrophy (Shy-Drager syndrome).

    Vascular: Basal ganglia infarction.

    Infectious: Postencephalitic.

The Depressed Auto Mechanic

Case 13

KEY TERMS

dystonia: Forceful, sustained contraction of a group of muscles.

palmomental reflex: A contraction of the superficial muscles of the chin produced on the same side as the palmar area that is stimulated (also called "palm-chin reflex").

glabellar reflex: A frontal release sign elicited by tapping the forehead repeatedly between the eyebrows over the glabella and by observing for persistent blinking. It is important to note that when this maneuver is performed, a normal individual will blink once or twice.

snout reflex: A frontal release sign elicited by repeatedly tapping the upper lip and by observing for puckering of the lips.

chorea: Irregular, unpredictable, and brief jerky movements that flit from one body part to another in a continuous, random sequence.

myoclonus: Spontaneous twitch of a group of muscles that moves a limb across a joint.

tic: Quick, stereotypic jerk of a group of facial or limb muscles.

phenothiazines: A chemical class of drugs used in a variety of psychotic disorders. Examples include chlorpromazine (Thorazine) and thioridazine (Mellaril).

HISTORY AND EXAMINATION

History of the Present Illness

A 40-year-old male automobile mechanic was referred to a neurologist for evaluation of involuntary movements. The patient relied on his wife to provide most of the history.

He first came to medical attention 2 years ago because of a suicide gesture. His family reports that he has had multiple extramarital sexual contacts over the past 10 years. He has a history of violent outbursts, especially at home. These have recently been interfering with his work. The family also reports that he has had marked emotional lability with periods of depression and apathy, one of which resulted in his previous suicide attempt. Over the past 6 months, his family has noted frequent jerking movements of his hands as well as pursing of his lips. The patient himself is oblivious to these movements. His internist was concerned by these findings and requested a neurological consultation.

Past Medical History

Depression with previous suicide attempt. In the past, he had been maintained on antidepressants and phenothiazines without clear benefit, although compliance with these drugs was a problem. There was a question of alcohol abuse in the past.

FAMILY HISTORY

His parents both died in an accident when he was 12 years old but were not known to have any health problems. He has a younger sister in good health. There is a vague history of a maternal aunt, "Crazy Aunt Irma," who died in a state hospital years ago. His own children are reportedly in good health, although his oldest daughter, who is 20 years of age, dropped out of college and has been much more withdrawn recently.

SOCIAL HISTORY

He is employed as an auto mechanic, a job he has held for the past 3 years. Previously, he owned and managed his own filling station but sold it because of financial difficulties and shrinking clientele. He reports no current use of alcohol or drugs.

Medications

None at present

Physical Examination

Slightly disheveled, initially guarded, and mildly hostile

Neurological Examination

On formal mental status testing, he remembered only two of three objects at 5 minutes and had poor calculation and visuospatial skills. His speech exhibited poor modulation of tone and volume. In addition, he had frequent grimacing and pursing movements of his mouth, as well as eyebrow elevation, especially while talking. He was quite demonstrative with his arms when he spoke but otherwise tended to rest his chin on his hands. When distracted he had involuntary, quick, irregular jerking movements of his fingers and hands and, to a lesser extent, of his feet. Occasionally he had some dystonic posturing of his neck and upper body. He had normal bulk and power in all four extremities. His sensory examination was normal. His reflexes were brisk, including the jaw jerk, and he had flexor plantar responses bilaterally. He had bilateral palmomental, glabellar, and snout reflexes. His gait was erratic, with some lurching.

Questions

1. What is the term applied to the involuntary movements exhibited by this patient?

2. List and define several other types of abnormal involuntary movements.

3. List five causes of chorea.

4. What movement disorders can you see with phenothiazines? Alcohol? Do phenothiazines and alcohol explain this patient's problems?

5. What is the most likely diagnosis for this patient? How can you verify it? Is this a genetically determined disease? If yes, what chromosome?

6. Is the patient's psychiatric history pertinent to his movement disorder?

7. Figure 35 compares the head computed tomography (CT) scan of this patient (A) with a head CT scan from a normal patient (B). What are the differences between these two scans?

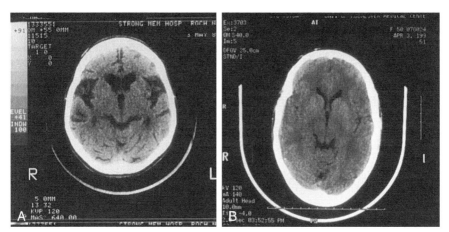

Figure 35. (A) Head CT scan from this patient. (B) Head CT scan from a normal individual.

8. What are treatments for chorea?

9. Should you be worried about the patient's eldest daughter?

Answers

1. What is the term applied to the involuntary movements exhibited by this patient?

   Chorea: Irregular, unpredictable, and brief jerky movements that flit from one body part to another in a continuous, random sequence.

2. List and define several other types of abnormal involuntary movements.

   Dyskinesia: Any movement disorder that displays excessive abnormal involuntary movements such as tremor, chorea, ballism, myoclonus, dystonia, tic, or athetosis.

   Tremor: Rhythmic oscillating movements resulting from alternating contractions of opposing muscle groups.

   Myoclonus: Spontaneous twitch of a group of muscles that moves a limb across a joint.

   Tic: Quick, stereotypical jerk of a group of facial or limb muscles.

   Athetosis: Slow, writhing, involuntary movements of the proximal limbs and trunk.

   Dystonia: Forceful, sustained contraction of a group of muscles.

   Hemiballism: Spontaneous, ballistic, irregular movements of the arm and leg on one side of the body.

3. List five causes of chorea.
   - Drug-induced (levodopa [L-dopa], cocaine, phenothiazines)
   - Neurodegenerative (Huntington's disease [HD], benign senile chorea)
   - Infectious (Sydenham's chorea—poststreptococcal)
   - Cerebral infarction (involving the basal ganglia)
   - Inflammatory (systemic lupus erythematosis, chorea gravidarum)

4. What movement disorders can you see with phenothiazines? Alcohol? Do phenothiazines and alcohol explain this patient's problems?

   Phenothiazines: A variety of movement disorders can be seen following the administration of phenothiazines, including dyskinesias, dystonia, akathisia, and parkinsonism. The onset of dyskinesia is often delayed 3 to 6 months after starting the phenothiazine, and this disorder is referred to as "tardive dyskinesia." "Akathisia" is motor restlessness, or the inability to sit still and the irresistible urge to move about.

Alcohol: Alcohol intoxication and withdrawal can cause a variety of movement disorders including tremor and chorea.

The progressive cognitive decline as well as the emerging personality disorder in this patient strongly indicates that the coexisting chorea is due to a neurodegenerative condition rather than solely to drug inducement.

5. What is the most likely diagnosis in this patient? How can you verify it? Is this a genetically determined disease? If yes, what chromosome?

The most likely diagnosis is Huntingdon's disease.

Traditionally, this diagnosis has been established by using clinical criteria, a positive family history, head CT scan showing atrophy of the head of the caudate nucleus, and genetic linkage analysis, if there are large numbers of involved family members. More recently, it has been possible to diagnose HD by analyzing the number of CAG trinucleotide repeats at the 5' end of the *HD* gene.

HD is an autosomal dominant disorder.

The abnormal gene, huntingtin, is found on chromosome 4.

6. Is the patient's psychiatric history pertinent to his movement disorder?

Yes. HD is a clinical triad of chorea, dementia, and psychosis.

7. Figure 35 compares the head CT scan of this patient (*A*) to a head CT scan from a normal patient (*B*). What are the differences between these two scans?

The patient's head CT scan (*A*) reveals atrophy of the head of the caudate nucleus, as well as generalized cortical atrophy.

8. What are treatments for chorea?

Dopamine receptor antagonists (e.g., phenothiazines) or dopamine-depleting agents (e.g., tetrabenazene, reserpine) may suppress chorea in the short term.

9. Should you be worried about the patient's eldest daughter?

Yes. This condition is inherited in an autosomal dominant fashion, and she may already be demonstrating a personality disorder.

The Ataxic Accountant

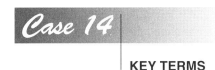

KEY TERMS

nystagmus: An involuntary rhythmic oscillation of the eyes.

internuclear ophthalmoplegia (INO): With attempted gaze to one side, failure of the adducting eye to move beyond the midline, with nystagmus developing in the abducting eye. INO is due to a lesion affecting the medial longitudinal fasciculus on the same side as the adducting eye.

optic disk: The area of the retina entered by the optic nerve.

Marcus Gunn pupil: A pupil that may react to light but does not hold the reaction, or, paradoxically, may dilate slowly; the consensual reflex may be more prompt than the direct reflex. These changes can often be brought about by rapid alternate stimulation of the eyes with bright light, a technique called the "swinging flashlight test." It is also referred to as an afferent pupillary defect.

evoked potential test: A diagnostic test in which electrical potentials are recorded from the scalp and result from a change in the ongoing electrical activity of neurons in response to stimulation of a sensory organ or pathway. Specific types of evoked potentials include visual evoked potentials, brain-stem auditory evoked potentials, and somatosensory evoked potentials.

oligoclonal bands: A particular electrophoresis staining pattern for cerebrospinal fluid (CSF) in patients with multiple sclerosis and other inflammatory conditions. In patients with normal cerebrospinal fluid, there is a homogenous agar gel staining in the immunoglobulin G (IgG) region. In patients with multiple sclerosis, the IgG region is heterogeneous, with the appearance of several distinctly staining bands, called oligoclonal bands.

HISTORY AND EXAMINATION

History of the Present Illness

C.R. is a 27-year-old woman who sees her physician because of dizziness and difficulty walking.

She was well until 7 years ago, when she had an episode of numbness in her legs, poor handwriting, and a staggering gait, which resolved spontaneously over a 3-week period. She was well for the next 5 years, when she again developed some mild difficulty in walking. Again, she improved on her own over a 2-week period and did well subsequently. She now presents with a 3-week history of such severe dizziness that it has caused her to fall several times. Over these past weeks, her walking has deteriorated steadily, and she must now hold onto furniture in order to get around her home. She also complains of double vision when looking off to her right side.

Past Medical History

She has never been seriously ill before. She has two healthy children, ages 5 and 3. She works part-time as an accountant. Her family history is unremarkable.

Medications

None

Physical Examination

She appears healthy. Her general examination is normal.

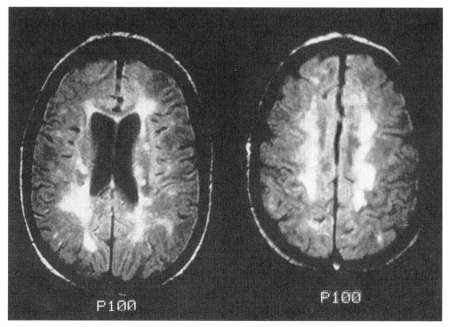

Figure 36. T1-weighted head MR scan with gadolinium contrast.

Neurological Examination

Her mental status is normal. On cranial nerve testing, the right optic disc appears paler than the left. Her ocular motility is normal on left gaze. However, when she looks to the right, the right eye develops some horizontal nystagmus, and the left eye does not completely adduct. On motor examination, muscle tone is increased in the lower extremities; muscle bulk and power are normal. Right ataxia is greater than left on finger-to-nose testing as well as on heel-to-shin testing. The sensory examination shows some loss of vibratory perception and proprioception at the toes. She sways when standing with her feet together, and swaying is made worse when she closes her eyes. Her reflexes are brisk throughout, with bilateral extensor plantar responses. She has a broad base when she walks and occasionally lurches to one side or the other. She is unable to perform a tandem gait.

A head magnetic resonance (MR) scan is performed and is shown in Figure 36.

Questions

1. How would you characterize the course of this patient's neurological disease?

2. What eye movement abnormality is being described? Where is the lesion? On which side?

3. Why do you think her right optic disc is pale? Although not explicitly stated in the examination, what would you predict her pupillary light reaction to reveal? What is the name for this pupillary light reaction?

4. List three lesions that cause broad-based gaits. Which do you think she has?

5. Where would you localize her lesion(s)?

6. Can all her abnormal findings be explained by a single lesion?

7. What is the most likely diagnosis? Why? What is the prognosis?

8. Figure 36 reveals the patient's MR scan. What features of this head MR scan help in making the diagnosis? Why are the lesions largely confined to the white matter?

9. Besides the head MR scan, what other diagnostic tests might be helpful in establishing the diagnosis?

10. What treatments are available?

11. Both Guillain-Barré syndrome and multiple sclerosis (MS) share a similar pathologic process. What is this process, and how do these diseases differ?

Answers

1. How would you characterize the course of this patient's neurological disease?

   She presents with relapsing and remitting neurological symptoms and signs.

2. What eye movement abnormality is being described? Where is the lesion? On which side?

   This patient has two important ocular motility abnormalities when looking to the right. First, when looking to the right, her left eye does not completely adduct (move toward the nose), and her right eye develops horizontal nystagmus. This combination of ocular signs is called an internuclear ophthalmoplegia (INO) and is caused by a lesion affecting the medial longitudinal fasciculus, which unites and coordinates the oculomotor and abducens nuclei. Because this patient has difficulty adducting her left eye, we can deduce that she has a lesion affecting her *left* medial longitudinal fasciculus (MLF) (See Fig. 27).

3. Why do you think her right optic disc is "pale"? Although not explicitly stated in the examination, what would you predict her pupillary light reaction to reveal? What is the name for this pupillary light reaction?

   A pale or atrophic optic disc suggests a history of optic neuritis. Patients with a history of optic neuritis will show abnormalities on pupillary light testing. Although the affected eye may react to direct light, it may not hold the reaction, or paradoxically, it may slowly dilate. The consensual reflex may be more prompt than the direct reflex and can be brought about by rapid alternate stimulation of the eyes with a bright light (the "swinging flashlight test"). This pupillary abnormality is called a Marcus Gunn pupil ("deafferented pupil") and is shown in Figure 37.

4. List three lesions that cause broad-based gaits. Which do you think she has?

Lesion Location	Abnormal Gait
Cerebellar vermis	Cerebellar ataxic gait
Dorsal columns of the spinal cord	Sensory ataxic gait
Bihemispheric disease	Gait apraxia

   Most likely, her gait disorder is a combination of both a cerebellar ataxic gait and a sensory ataxic gait. The wide-based and lurching quality of her gait is characteristic of cerebellar disease, whereas the augmentation of her unsteadiness (mani-

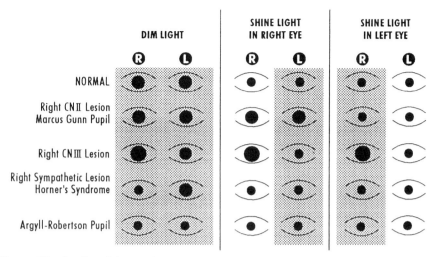

Figure 37. Pupillary light reactions.

fested as increased swaying) when she closes her eyes is due to the loss of proprioception in her lower extremities.

5. Where would you localize her lesion(s)?

Sign or Symptom	Lesion
Pale optic disc	Right optic nerve
Internuclear ophthalmoplegia	An MLF lesion within the brain stem
Ataxia	Brain stem, cerebellum, or spinal cord
Hyperrflexia, spasticity, Babinski's sign	Cerebral white matter
Large-fiber sensory loss	Dorsal columns of spinal cord
Romberg's sign	Dorsal columns of spinal cord

6. Can all her abnormal findings be explained by a single lesion?
   No. She has more than one lesion, as noted above.

7. What is the most likely diagnosis? Why? What is the prognosis?
   Diagnosis: Multiple sclerosis. She has more than one lesion and at least one previous episode. This illustrates dispersion of lesions in time and space, which is the crucial criterion for diagnosing MS.
   Prognosis: Variable. Her course may continue to be relapsing and remitting, she may stabilize, or she may develop the chronic progressive form of the disease.

8. What features of the head MR scan (Fig. 36) help in making the diagnosis? Why are the lesions largely confined to the white matter?

This head MR scan demonstrates multiple areas of high-signal abnormalities (bright areas) in the centrum semiovale and periventricular white matter. These represent a mixture of acute and chronic demyelinating plaques.

The lesions on MR are primarily in the white matter because most myelin is located in the white matter.

9. Besides the head MR scan, what other diagnostic tests might be helpful in establishing the diagnosis?

Other diagnostic tests include visual evoked responses (VERs) and brain-stem auditory evoked responses (BAERs). These studies assess the integrity of nerve conduction through the visual (VERs) and auditory (BAERs) pathways. Any demyelinating plaques along these pathways will slow nerve conduction. This slowing can be detected by comparing it to normative data or the velocities recorded on the contralateral side.

An additional diagnostic test could include a lumbar puncture with CSF analysis. In patients with MS, the CSF may demonstrate abnormal central nervous system (CNS) protein synthesis, which is identified by oligoclonal banding and an elevated IgG index.

10. What treatments are available?

High-dose intravenous corticosteroids for acute exacerbation (symptomatic therapy).

Three immune-modulating agents are currently available for patients with relapsing remitting MS: interferon β-1b (Betaseron), interferon β-1a (Avonex), and glatiramer acetate (Copaxone). These agents move beyond the traditional symptomatic therapies and appear to fundamentally alter the course of MS.

For patients with chronic progressive MS, immunosuppressive agents such as azathioprine and cyclophosphamide are often used.

11. Both Guillain-Barré syndrome and MS share a similar pathologic process. What is this process, and how do these diseases differ?

The common process is demyelination. Guillain-Barré syndrome is an *acute* monophasic illness and is associated with *peripheral nervous system* demyelination. MS is a *chronic* disease with exacerbations and remissions and is associated with *central nervous system* demyelination.

The Unsteady Bookkeeper

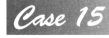

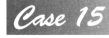

| KEY TERMS

vertigo: The sensation of moving around in space or of having objects move about the person.

hypertension: A condition in which the patient has a higher than normal blood pressure.

intention tremor: A tremor exhibited or intensified when attempting coordinated movements.

supple neck: No pain or discomfort on passive flexion and extension of the neck.

lipohyalinosis: The neuropathologic changes noted in the small arteries that result in small cerebral infarctions.

lumbar puncture: A puncture made by placing an aspiration needle into the subarachnoid space of the spinal cord, usually in the lumbar area at the level of the fourth intervertebral space to sample cerebrospinal fluid (CSF) for analysis.

HISTORY AND EXAMINATION

History of the Present Illness

A.K. is a 62-year-old woman who is brought to the emergency room by her friend because of dizziness and difficulty walking.

A.K. took a nap the evening before admission, and when she awoke later that evening, she experienced some nausea, dizziness, and vertigo. She arose and walked carefully to the bathroom, holding onto the furniture and walls. In the bathroom, she vomited once and then fell asleep sitting on the commode. She slept there overnight and awoke the next morning with a bifrontal headache and continued nausea and dizziness. She therefore called a friend, who took her to the emergency room.

Past Medical History

She has a history of hypertension for the past 15 years and exertional angina for the past 5 years. She works as a bookkeeper for a local fuel oil company.

Medications

β-blocker for hypertension. Nitroglycerin tablets as needed for chest pain.

Physical Examination

She is moderately obese. BP = 200/130 mm Hg; P = 76/min. She presents no evidence of head trauma, and her neck is supple. There is a soft

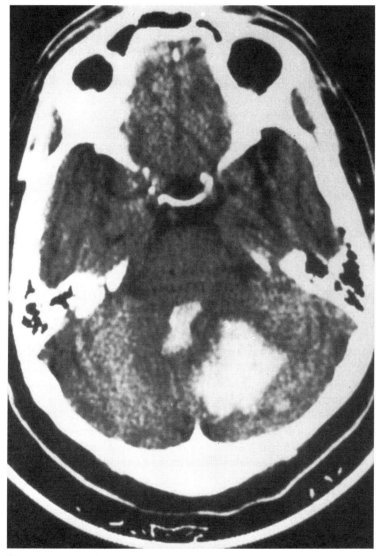

Figure 38. Head CT scan, without contrast.

systolic murmur along the left ventricular outflow tract, and there are no carotid bruits.

Neurological Examination

She is sleepy but answers questions appropriately. Her fundi reveal flat optic discs with some copper wiring. Her pupils are equal and symmetrically reactive to light. On extraocular muscle testing, she has some nystagmus on right gaze. On motor testing, some decreased muscle tone in the right arm and leg is noticeable, but her bulk and strength are normal. Intention tremor was found on right finger-to-nose and heel-to-shin testing. Sensory testing is normal. Her reflexes are normoactive and symmetrical, and she has an extensor plantar response on the left. Her gait is broad-based, and she lists toward the right side. She is unable to perform a tandem gait.

A head computed tomography (CT) scan is emergently obtained (Fig. 38).

Questions

1. Name the areas of the nervous system that, when damaged, cause a decrease in muscle tone (hypotonia). Why is her muscle tone decreased on the right side?

2. Describe the major inputs and outputs of the cerebellum, and indicate where these fiber tracts cross. Do cerebellar lesions produce ipsilateral or contralateral symptoms? Why?

3. Why did she develop vertigo, nausea, and dizziness? Headache?

4. Her head CT is shown in Figure 38. A pathologic specimen from a patient who died from a similar condition is shown in Figure 39. What do you think is the etiology of her lesion?

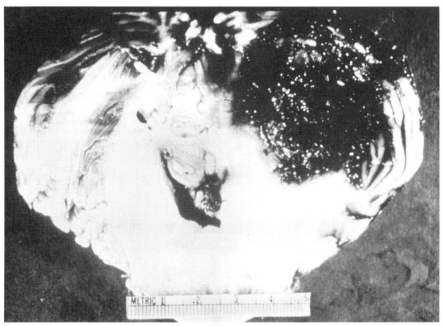

Figure 39.   Gross specimen from a patient who died from a condition similar to that shown in Figure 38.

5. Hemorrhage into the brain is one type of stroke. Define stroke, and list other causes of stroke.

6. What role does hypertension have in her illness?

7. What other areas of the brain are susceptible to the same type of stroke experienced by A.K.? What neurological symptoms would lesions in these areas produce?

8. Why is CT superior to magnetic resonance (MR) in this clinical setting?

9. If the patient were to become lethargic, what do you think might be going on?

10. Why should a lumbar puncture *not* be performed in this patient?

11. What is the prognosis? What is the treatment?

Answers

1. Name the areas of the nervous system that, when damaged, cause a decrease in muscle tone (hypotonia). Why is her muscle tone decreased on the right side?

   The cerebellum helps to regulate muscle tone and when the cerebellum is lesioned, muscle tone is decreased. Lower motor neuron lesions also result in decreased muscle tone. An acute upper motor neuron lesion can also cause transient hypotonia (See Case 7).

   A right cerebellar lesion (suggested by the right-sided ataxia) would cause decreased muscle tone on that side.

2. Describe the major inputs and outputs of the cerebellum, and indicate where these fiber tracts cross. Do cerebellar lesions produce ipsilateral or contralateral symptoms? Why?

Peduncle	Inputs	Outputs
Superior	Ventral spinocerebellar tracts	Red nucleus
	Superior and inferior colliculi	Ventral lateral nucleus of thalamus
	Trigeminal system	
Middle	Corticopontine fibers	
Inferior	Dorsal and rostral spinocerebellar tracts	Vestibular nuclei
	Cuneocerebellar tract	Reticular formation
	Inferior olive	
	Vestibular nuclei	
	Reticular formation	

Crossings: All inputs are uncrossed except for the ventral spinocerebellar tract, which crosses twice: in the spinal cord and in the midbrain (at the decussation of the superior cerebellar peduncle).

All outputs via the superior cerebellar peduncle cross on exit.

Cerebellar lesions produce ipsilateral deficits because the inputs are ipsilateral, and the outputs effectively cross twice: in the midbrain (Figs. 40 and 41) and at the medullary pyramids (not shown), where the corticospinal motor output crosses.

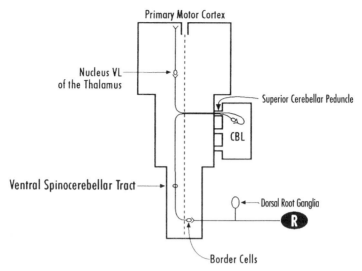

Figure 40. Spinocerebellar pathways: ventral spinocerebellar tract. CBL = cerebellum, R = receptor, VL = ventral lateral.

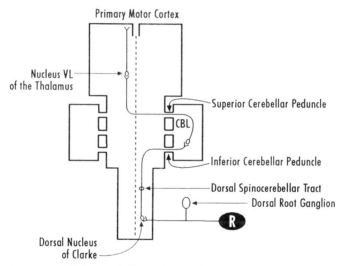

Figure 41. Spinocerebellar pathways: dorsal spinocerebellar tract. CBL = cerebullum, R = receptor, VL = ventral lateral.

3. Why did she develop vertigo, nausea, and dizziness? Headache?

Vertigo, nausea, and dizziness are due to pressure on the brain-stem vestibular nuclei in the pons and medulla.

Acute strokes can cause headaches, particularly if they occur in the posterior fossa and are associated with increased intracranial pressure. Intracerebral hemorrhages cause headaches more often than ischemic strokes do.

4. Her head CT is shown in Figure 38. A pathologic specimen from a patient who died from a similar condition is shown in Figure 39. What do you think is the etiology of her lesion?

The noncontrasted head CT scan shown in Figure 38 reveals a large area of acute hemorrhage into the left cerebellar hemisphere. Blood is also seen in the fourth ventricle. Figure 39 shows a massive clot of blood occupying the right cerebellar hemisphere, with extension into the subarachnoid space over the folia of both hemispheres. One can also see distortion and displacement of the fourth ventricle and vermis to the opposite side as a consequence of the blood clot and edema of the affected hemisphere.

Hypertension is the most common etiology for an intracerebral hemorrhage. Given her past history of hypertension and her elevated blood pressure on examination (200/130 mm Hg), it is the likely cause of her intracerebral hemorrhage.

5. Hemorrhage into the brain is one type of stroke. Define stroke, and list other causes of stroke.

Stroke: A neurological deficit of sudden onset due to a pathologic process involving intracerebral blood vessels.

Causes of Stroke
- Ischemic (embolic, small- or large-vessel thrombotic, vasculitic, arterial dissection) (See Case 6)
- Hemorrhagic (intraparenchymal, subarachnoid)
- Migraine with aura (complicated migraine)

6. What role does hypertension have in her illness?

Hypertension causes lipohyalinosis of small penetrating intracerebral arterioles, which predisposes the patient to intracerebral hemorrhage.

7. What other areas of the brain are susceptible to the same type of stroke experienced by A.K.? What neurological symptoms would lesions in these areas produce?

Lesion Location	Signs or Symptoms
Basal ganglia	Contralateral hemiparesis due to compression of internal capsule
Pons	Brain-stem dysfunction "Pinpoint" pupils Ophthalmoplegia

Thalamus	Contralateral hemisensory loss
Gray–white-matter junction	Lobar (hemispheric) signs (e.g., contralateral hemiparesis, or homonymous hemianopia, aphasia, apraxia, and agnosia)

8. Why is CT superior to MR in this clinical setting?

   CT is excellent in detecting acute bleeding.

9. If the patient were to become lethargic, what do you think might be going on?

   She may be developing brain-stem compression, which may lead to cerebellar tonsillar herniation as well as an obstructive, noncommunicating hydrocephalus.

10. Why should a lumbar puncture *not* be performed in this patient?

    A lumbar puncture may accelerate herniation of the cerebellar tonsils through the foramen magnum. Herniation occurs because a lumbar puncture decreases intraspinal pressure, thereby increasing the pressure differential between the posterior fossa and the spinal canal.

11. What is the prognosis? What is the treatment?

    Prognosis: Good, if she does not develop severe posterior fossa edema.

    Treatment: Close observation. Neurosurgical evaluation for posterior fossa decompression, ventriculostomy, or both if she deteriorates clinically.

The Numb Ballroom Dancer

KEY TERMS

dysesthesia: Perverted interpretations of sensations, such as a burning or tingling feeling in response to tactile or painful stimulation.

neglect: Lack of attention or unresponsiveness to stimuli presented on the side opposite a damaged brain hemisphere.

sensory drift: Profound loss of sensation can cause a "sensory drift" resulting in an inability to localize in space. This does not represent a pronator drift (pronation, abduction, and internal rotation), which is specific to upper motor neuron dysfunction.

electrocardiogram (ECG): A record of the electrical activity of the heart.

thalamic pain syndrome (syndrome of Déjérine-Roussy): Distressing spontaneous pain and discomfort on the side of the body opposite a lesion (usually vascular) involving the ventroposterolateral (VPL) and ventroposteromedial (VPM) nuclei of the thalamus.

HISTORY AND EXAMINATION

History of the Present Illness

A 54-year-old, right-handed ballroom dancer presents to the emergency room complaining that her left side "does not feel right." The symptoms started 11 hours previously in her left hand while she was dancing at a party; within 90 minutes, they involved her entire left side. She presently states that she "cannot feel a thing" on her left side. She is clumsy with her left hand and has difficulty walking. She reports no headache, diplopia, vertigo, or visual symptoms. Three days ago, she had a transient 10-minute episode of paresthesias in her left arm. Although she found this peculiar, she brought it to no one's attention.

Past Medical History

Mild essential hypertension for the past 6 years

Medications

None. She never took antihypertensive medication.

Physical Examination

BP = 167/98 mm Hg; P = 76/min, regular; R = 14/min; afebrile. She is extremely pleasant and in no distress. There are no carotid bruits or cardiac murmurs.

Neurological Examination

Mental status is normal with intact language and visuospatial skills (she drew a clock and a three-dimensional cube). She demonstrates no left-sided neglect. On cranial nerve testing, her pupils are 5/5 mm and react briskly to 3/3 mm. Her visual fields are full to confrontation. Her ocular motility is full, without nystagmus. She has profound sensory loss to all modalities over her entire left head. When tested with a pin, coursing from the left scalp to her right, she yells "now" consistently when the pin reaches the midline. Her corneal reflexes are brisk bilaterally. Her face is symmetrical and strong. On motor testing, she has normal tone and bulk. On formal testing, she has grade 5 strength throughout. With her eyes closed and her arms held outstretched and pronated, her left arm randomly wanders in space, drifting in all directions. She is grossly ataxic on left finger-to-nose and heel-to-shin testing. Profound left hemibody sensory loss is present. She

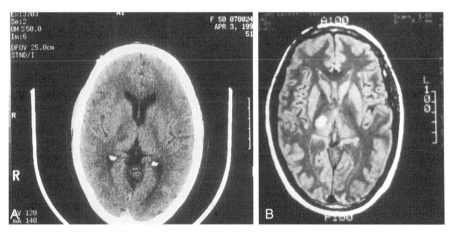

Figure 42. *(A)* Head CT scan; *(B)* proton density MR scan from the same patient. Note that the patient's right is on the left side of both images.

perceives only a vague light touch when her left side is touched. Her muscle stretch reflexes are symmetrical and normal throughout. Her plantar responses are flexor bilaterally. Her gait is unsteady.

You order a head computed tomography (CT). Two days later, she starts experiencing dysesthesias in her left arm, and you order a head magnetic resonance (MR) scan (Fig. 42).

Questions

1. List at least three regions in the neuraxis that, if lesioned, can produce a left hemibody sensory loss.

2. In this patient, what is the importance of the absence of left-sided neglect?

3. Why does her left arm wander in space when her eyes are closed? Does this represent a pronator drift?

4. Localize this woman's lesion.

5. What is the vascular supply to the involved territory in this patient?

6. Figure 42 shows her head CT and proton-density MR scan. What is the likely etiology of her lesion?

7. What role does hypertension have in her illness?

8. What further investigation and treatment do you recommend?

9. What syndrome is she at risk for developing?

Answers

1. List at least three regions in the neuraxis that, if lesioned, can produce a left hemibody sensory loss?
   - Right parietal cortex
   - Right corona radiata
   - Right thalamus
   - Right dorsal pons

2. In this patient, what is the importance of the absence of left-sided neglect?

   The ability to attend to a hemispatial field is a function of the contralateral parietal lobe. Because she does not have neglect, the lesion is not likely to be in the right parietal cortex.

3. Why does her left arm wander in space when her eyes are closed? Does this represent a pronator drift?

   Profound loss of sensation can cause a "sensory drift" resulting in an inability to localize in space. This does not represent a pronator drift (pronation, abduction, and internal rotation), which is specific to upper motor neuron dysfunction. (See Case 7.)

4. Localize this woman's lesion.

   Profound hemisensory lesions that split the midline are often seen in lesions of the thalamus, where the sensory inputs converge. Her lesion localizes to the right thalamus in the lateral and medial division of the ventral posterior nuclei (VPL and VPM) (Figs. 43–46). These sensory relay nuclei relay somatosensory and facial sensory information to the primary sensory cortex.

5. What is the vascular supply to the involved territory in this patient?

   Thalamogeniculate branches off the right posterior cerebral artery.

6. Figure 42 shows her head CT and proton-density MR scan. What is the likely etiology of her lesion?

   The head MR scan (*B*) shows a well-circumscribed high-signal (bright) lesion in the right lateral thalamus in the region of the VPL and VPM nuclei. In a similar location to the lesion identified on the head MR scan, the head CT scan (*A*) shows a well-circumscribed area of decreased density.

   The most likely etiology is a small cerebral infarct (lacunar infarct) from small-vessel disease. (See also Case 9.)

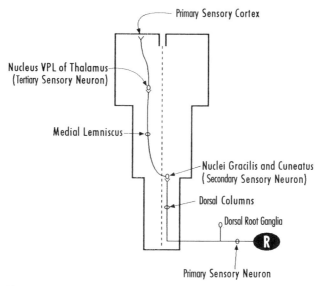

Figure 43. The proprioception-vibration sensory pathways. R = receptor, VPL = ventral posterolateral.

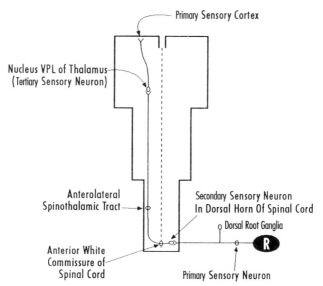

Figure 44. The pain-temperature sensory pathways. R = receptor, VPL = ventral posterolateral.

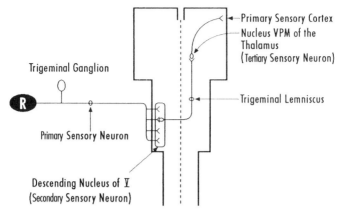

Figure 45. Trigeminal pain-temperature sensory system. R = receptor, VPM = ventral posteromedial.

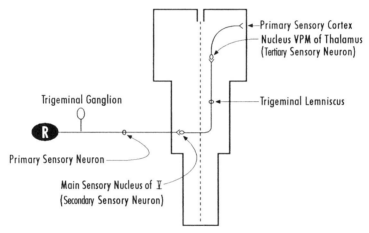

Figure 46. Trigeminal proprioception-vibration sensory system. R = receptor, VPM = ventral posteromedial.

7. What role does hypertension have in her illness?

   A long-standing history of hypertension is a major risk factor for the development of small-vessel cerebrovascular disease. Diabetes mellitus is also a risk factor for small-vessel cerebrovascular disease.

8. What further investigation and treatment do you recommend?

   Further testing: ECG, transesophageal echocardiography, serum cholesterol, and a serum glucose.

   Treatment: Hypertension control, aspirin 325 mg/day; correct other modifiable risk factors, if present.

9. What syndrome is she at risk for developing?

   Thalamic pain syndrome (syndrome of Déjérine-Roussy): Involvement of the VPL and VPM nuclei of the thalamus, which is usually due to a vascular lesion, can give rise to distressing spontaneous pain and discomfort on the side contralateral to the lesion.

The Insensitive Graduate Student

KEY TERMS

lymphadenopathy: A disease of the lymph nodes.

small-fiber neuropathy: Neuropathy that preferentially affects the pain-temperature pathway; neuropathies that preferentially affect the proprioception-vibration sensory pathway are referred to as large-fiber neuropathies.

HISTORY AND EXAMINATION

History of the Present Illness

A 25-year-old graduate student is seen by a neurologist because of tingling in his hands and feet.

The sensations in his feet began about 6 months ago, but he recently noticed that his fingers began to feel numb and tingle as well. When he steps into the shower, he notices that he cannot feel the temperature of the water with his feet. He has had no trouble with balance or walking in the dark. Occasionally the soles of his feet "burn" at night, and it is hard for him to fall asleep because of the burning.

In addition, he has lost about 15 pounds unintentionally. He blames this on a decreased appetite due to his intravenous (IV) cocaine habit, which he feels helps increase his productivity.

Past Medical History

Otherwise unremarkable

Medications

None

Physical Examination

T = 37°C; BP = 110/60 mm Hg; P = 88/min. He is thin and appears ill. He has palpably enlarged cervical, axillary, and inguinal lymph nodes.

Neurological Examination

His mental status and cranial nerves are normal. Motor examination reveals normal bulk, tone, and power. Light touch, pin, and temperature sensations are significantly decreased from the knees distally and in the finger tips. There is a slightly decreased vibratory sensation at the toes. Reflexes are absent at the ankles, trace at the knees, and normal in the upper extremities. Plantar responses are flexor bilaterally. His gait is wide-based and slightly unsteady.

Questions

1. Where along the neuraxis would you localize this patient's lesion?

2. What is the significance of this patient's history of IV drug abuse? His weight loss? His lymphadenopathy?

3. How does this case differ from Case 16 with respect to the neuroanatomic structure primarily involved?

4. What is meant by *large-fiber* and *small-fiber neuropathy*? What type of neuropathy does this patient have? Why are pain and temperature sensation more affected than vibration?

5. What is meant by a *dying-back neuropathy*, and why does it often lead to a stocking-glove distribution of sensory loss?

6. What is Romberg's test? Would you expect it to be abnormal in this patient?

7. What is the most likely etiology of his problem, and what could be done to help him?

8. What other neurological complications can be seen in this disorder?

Answers

1. Where along the neuraxis would you localize this patient's lesion?

   In the peripheral nerves, owing to the fact that he has hyporeflexia and distal sensory loss.

2. What is the significance of this patient's history of IV drug abuse? His weight loss? His lymphadenopathy?

   Intravenous drug abuse: A risk factor for acquiring the human immunodeficiency virus (HIV).

   Weight loss and adenopathy: Constitutional symptoms suggesting progression of the HIV infection.

3. How does this case differ from Case 16 with respect to the neuroanatomic structure primarily involved?

   The sensory disturbance in this patient stems from disease in the peripheral nervous system. Disease in the central nervous system (CNS) was seen in Case 16.

4. What is meant by *large-fiber* and *small-fiber neuropathy*? What type of neuropathy does this patient have? Why are pain and temperature sensation more affected than vibration?

   The primary sensory neurons of the pain-temperature sensory pathways are anatomically smaller than the primary sensory neurons of the proprioception-vibration sensory pathway. Therefore, those neuropathies that preferentially affect the pain-temperature pathway are often referred to as *small-fiber neuropathies*, whereas those neuropathies that preferentially affect the proprioception-vibration sensory pathway are referred to as *large-fiber neuropathies*. In this patient, pain and temperature are more severely involved than proprioception-vibration, and hence, his neuropathy is more consistent with a small-fiber neuropathy.

5. What is meant by *dying-back neuropathy*, and why does it often lead to a stocking-glove distribution of sensory loss?

   Dying-back neuropathy is seen in most toxic neuropathies; it is a neuropathy that occurs when a toxin purportedly interferes with protein synthesis, which occurs solely in the neuronal cell body. This leads to degeneration of the most distal segments of the longest axons (*length-dependent vulnerability*), resulting in this characteristic pattern of sensory loss. The disease process is fiber-length dependent and, therefore, the longest nerve fibers are affected first in their most peripheral segments (i.e., in the distal feet and hands). This pattern of sensory loss is often referred to as *stocking-glove distribution of sensory dysfunction.*

6. What is Romberg's test? Would you expect it to be abnormal in this patient?

Romberg's test is a functional test of the sensory system and is performed by asking the patient to stand with his or her feet together and eyes closed. The patient is then observed to see if balance can be maintained. The test is positive if the patient falls to one side. Because this patient has defective proprioception, his Romberg's test would probably be positive.

7. What is the most likely etiology of his problem, and what could be done to help him?

Etiology: HIV-related sensory neuropathy.

Symptomatic treatment: Low-dose tricyclic antidepressants can be used for pain control. A treatment regimen of HIV reverse transcriptase inhibitors and protease inhibitors may reduce mortality and delay progression of disease.

8. What other neurological complications can be seen in this disorder?

Process	Complication
Primary HIV infection	HIV dementia
	Vacuolar myelopathy
	HIV myopathy
Opportunistic infections	CNS toxoplasmosis
	Cytomegalovirus encephalitis and polyradiculitis
	Progressive multifocal leukoencephalopathy
	Cryptococcal meningitis
Malignancies	Primary CNS lymphoma

The Retired Cat Burglar

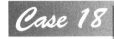

KEY TERMS

corneal reflex: Closure of eyelids resulting from direct corneal irritation.

Weber test: The use of a tuning fork to distinguish between unilateral sensorineural and conduction deafness.

Rinne test: The use of a tuning fork to compare bone conduction hearing with air conduction hearing.

brain-stem auditory evoked response (BAER): The study of brain waves during sound stimuli as determined by a method independent of the individual's subjective response.

audiogram: A graphic record of sound perception produced by an audiometer.

HISTORY AND EXAMINATION

History of the Present Illness

M.B. is a 43-year-old retired cat burglar. He had been effectively applying his trade for many years when he noted the slow onset of hearing loss in the left ear. This was not a major problem at first, as long as he was attentive with his good ear. Just before his retirement, he began to notice an odd sensation of fullness in the back of his head. From time to time, he would also become unsteady when walking, especially after a quick turn. He also noted mild problems with his balance and agility. On the night of his retirement, he failed to hear an alarm because of a hissing noise that had become progressively worse in his left ear. When he became aware of the police department's presence, he made for a quick window exit. On stooping over and turning to exit through the window, however, he noted the acute onset of dizziness and lost his balance. He fell a short distance from the window to a roof rather noisily and was retired to the city lockup.

Past Medical History

Unremarkable

Medications

None

Physical Examination

On examination downtown, the patient related his recent problems with hearing and balance, especially with turning, to an interested medical student. His tympanic membranes appeared normal bilaterally.

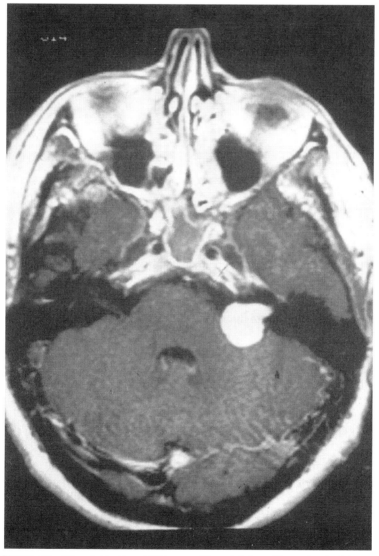

Figure 47. T1-weighted head MR scan with gadolinium. The patient's right side is on the left side of the image.

Neurological Examination

Although most of his examination was normal, the medical student found that there was a definite hearing loss on the left, with poor speech discrimination and decreased perception of loud noises. A tuning fork placed at the vertex of the head was louder for him in the right ear. The corneal reflexes were as follows:

Right: Direct—normal; consensual—depressed.

Left: Direct—depressed; consensual—normal.

Facial sensation appeared normal. His left face was mildly weak compared with the right. She found no other definite abnormalities on examination.

Two days later, a head magnetic resonance (MR) scan was obtained (Fig. 47).

Questions

1. What can cause unilateral hearing loss?

2. What did this patient imply when he said he was dizzy? What are other possible causes of "dizziness"?

3. Which neurological systems are necessary to maintain balance?

4. How does poor speech discrimination help you in localizing his lesion?

5. Would you expect this patient to have problems closing his left eye tightly? If yes, why; if not, why not?

6. What is the Weber test? The Rinne test? How do these tests help in further evaluating hearing deficits?

7. Describe the neuroanatomic pathway for the corneal reflex. Describe what you would see when the right corneal reflex was elicited in this patient. How would the findings differ if he had left-sided facial sensory loss and no facial weakness?

8. What does his T1-weighted head MR scan with gadolinium (Fig. 47) show? What is the most likely etiology of his lesion?

9. What would you expect his BAER to show? His audiogram?

Answers

1. What can cause unilateral hearing loss?

    Any disease process affecting the middle or inner ear apparatus or the eighth cranial nerve may cause deafness. Examples include:
    - Otitis media
    - Otosclerosis (hardening of the ossicles)
    - Ménière's disease
    - Presbyacusis (high-frequency hearing loss in the elderly)
    - Acoustic schwannoma

2. What did this patient imply when he said he was dizzy? What are other possible causes of "dizziness"?

    Dizziness is a nonspecific symptom and means many different things to different patients. When patients complain of "dizziness", it is important to query them further to obtain a more accurate description and etiology of their symptoms. This patient probably was experiencing vertigo because of the positional nature of his symptoms and the associated hearing loss.
    Other causes of "dizziness":
    - Syncope and presyncope
    - Defective proprioception (disequilibrium)
    - Diplopia with visual disorientation
    - Hyperventilation-induced lightheadedness

3. Which neurological systems are necessary to maintain balance?

    Several neurological systems assist in the proper maintenance of balance. These systems include the proprioception-vibration system (dorsal column pathways), the visual system, and the vestibular-midline cerebellum system. Balance can be impaired if there is abrupt loss to one system, such as the vestibular–midline cerebellum system affected in this patient, or a chronic slow impairment of all systems, as seen in many elderly patients. Compensation can occur; for example, many legally blind patients are not "off-balance" because the other two systems have compensated for the loss of vision and its role in maintaining balance.

4. How does poor speech discrimination help you in localizing his lesion?

    To test for speech discrimination, the patient is asked to repeat a series of monosyllabic words that are presented at suprathreshold intensity. The percentage of words repeated correctly is recorded.

Speech discrimination is preserved in patients with a sensorineural hearing loss, which is cochlear in origin. Poor speech discrimination is seen with lesions of the cochlear nerve or more rostral parts of the auditory pathway (e.g., lateral lemniscus fibers or the inferior colliculi) (Fig. 48).

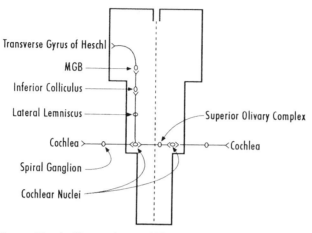

Figure 48. Auditory pathways. MGB = medial geniculate body.

5. Would you expect this patient to have problems closing his left eye tightly? If yes, why; if not, why not?

Yes, because he has a facial nerve (peripheral cranial VII) lesion resulting in left facial weakness.

6. What is the Weber test? The Rinne test? How do these tests help in further evaluating hearing deficits?

Weber test: A tuning fork (512 Hz) placed on the vertex of the head is normally heard equally in each ear and does not lateralize (Fig. 49). In patients with sensorineural deafness, the tuning fork lateralizes to (i.e., is heard better in) the "good" ear. In patients with conduction deafness, the tuning fork lateralizes to the affected ear.

Rinne test: The base of a tuning fork (512 Hz) is placed on the mastoid process (bone conduction) (Fig. 49). When the sound ceases, the tines of the fork are placed adjacent to the auditory meatus (air conduction) and the patient is asked if he or she still hears the sound. A normal response occurs when air conduction is louder than bone conduction (also true in sensorineural hearing loss). An abnormal response occurs when bone conduction is louder than air conduction, suggesting a conductive hearing loss.

Weber Test

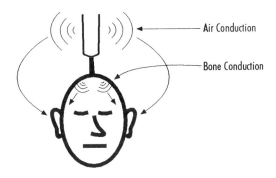

Rinne Test

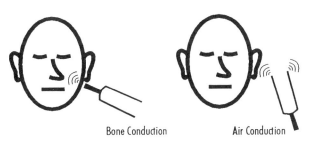

Bone Conduction   Air Conduction

Figure 49. The Weber test and the Rinne test.

7. Describe the neuroanatomic pathway for the corneal reflex. Describe what you would see when the right corneal reflex was elicited in this patient. How would the findings differ if he had left-sided facial sensory loss and no facial weakness?

    Corneal reflex: Afferent loop—trigeminal nerve; efferent loop—facial nerve (Fig. 50).

    Testing of the right corneal reflex in this patient would show a normal blink response on the right but not on the left.

    If the patient had left-sided facial sensory loss and no facial weakness, the findings would be:

    Right: Direct—normal response; consensual—normal response.

    Left: Direct—depressed response; consensual—depressed response.

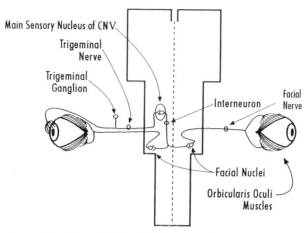

Figure 50. Corneal reflex. This is an excellent way to test the sensory component of the trigeminal nerve, as well as the facial nerve. To test this reflex, the cornea is touched with a wisp of cotton and the resultant direct and consensual eye blinks are noted. The afferent information of this reflex is carried by the ophthalmic division of the trigeminal nerve, and the efferent information is carried by the facial nerve.

8. What does his T1-weighted head MR scan with gadolinium (Fig. 47) show? What is the most likely etiology of his lesion?

The MR scan shows a well-circumscribed enhancing lesion without surrounding edema extending from the internal auditory canal into the left cerebello-pontine angle.

Most likely, this represents an acoustic schwannoma.

9. What would you expect his BAER to show? His audiogram?

BAER: The stimulation of an ear evokes a characteristic response that can be detected by brain-stem auditory evoked potentials. There are seven potentials or waves that show an electrophysiological-anatomic correlation. Wave I and wave II correspond to the auditory nerve and the cochlear nucleus (in pons), respectively. Therefore, an acoustic schwannoma delaying conduction of auditory nerve would cause a prolongation in the interlatency difference between waves I and II on the left side.

Audiogram: Sensorineural hearing loss in the left ear.

The Spinning Pastry Maker

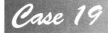

KEY TERMS

tinnitus: A ringing sound in the ear.

peripheral vertigo: Vertigo due to disturbances in the vestibular apparatus of the inner ear.

central vertigo: Vertigo caused by disease of the central nervous system.

conductive hearing loss: Hearing loss resulting from a lesion to structures in the outer or middle ear that converts air conduction into bone conduction.

sensorineural hearing loss: Hearing loss resulting from a lesion involving the inner ear (cochlear apparatus) or the eighth cranial nerve.

saccades: Fast, voluntary movements of the eyes as they change from one point of gaze to another.

electronystagmogram (ENG): A record of nystagmus activity, measured by detecting the electrical activity of the extraocular muscles.

HISTORY AND EXAMINATION

History of the Present Illness

Ms. W.F. is a 45-year-old pastry maker who noted recent problems with her hearing. An avid tea drinker, she noted that she was having trouble hearing her kettle. At times she heard whistling in her ears that was not produced by the kettle; at other times she could not hear the kettle when it did whistle. This went on for several months, getting gradually worse in both ears. One morning while getting out of bed, she began to hear whistling again, which became progressively louder. As it was becoming annoying, she suddenly felt the room begin to spin. She sat back down, but sitting gave her no relief; she became nauseated and eventually vomited. Because the spinning persisted, she climbed back in bed and found herself to be more comfortable when she lay on her right

151

side with her eyes open. Within half an hour, the spinning had abated, and after that, the whistling also diminished.

Since then, she has had several more similar episodes, each beginning with increasing whistling followed by a spinning sensation. Mild hearing problems and baseline whistling in both ears persist as well. Between her attacks she feels quite well and has no difficulty with her strength or coordination. She has taken to heating water for her tea in her microwave.

Past Medical History

Unremarkable

Medications

None

Physical Examination

She appears well. The general examination is unremarkable.

Neurological Examination

Her mental status is normal. She has bilateral hearing loss with relative preservation of speech discrimination. She also complains of whistling in her ears. The other cranial nerves as well as the rest of the neurological examination are normal.

Although she was well through most of the examination, near the end she noted increasing whistling and had a mild attack of this spinning sensation. During that attack, nystagmus was noted with fast beating to the right. The spinning, whistling, and nystagmus abated before she left.

Questions

1. What is vertigo?

2. How does vertigo from a central (brain stem) cause differ clinically from peripheral vertigo (due to vestibular organ dysfunction)?

3. What is tinnitus? What are the two different types of tinnitus?

4. What is a conductive hearing loss? A sensorineural hearing loss? How can the two be differentiated, both by history and physical findings, and with laboratory studies?

5. This patient felt more comfortable during her vertiginous attack when she lay on her right side. How does this fact help you to localize her lesion?

6. Nystagmus with the fast-beating component to the right suggests vestibular dysfunction on which side? Why?

7. Given the symptom complex, what is the most likely diagnosis? What further tests would be helpful?

8. How would you treat this patient?

Answers

1. What is vertigo?

   Vertigo: A sensation of motion of self or surroundings.

2. How does vertigo from a central (brain stem) cause differ clinically from peripheral vertigo (due to vestibular organ dysfunction)?

Central Vertigo	Peripheral Vertigo
Vertigo is mild	Vertigo is severe
Brain-stem signs are present	No brain-stem signs are present
Hearing loss is rare	Hearing loss is common
Nystagmus is:	Nystagmus is:
Multidirectional	Unidirectional
Nonfatigable	Fatigable
Abrupt in onset	Of long latency of onset
Of long duration	Of short duration

5. What is tinnitus? What are the two different types of tinnitus?

   Tinnitus: The perception of abnormal sounds in the ear. The sounds are most often ringing but may be buzzing, humming, whistling, roaring, hissing, clicking, or pulselike.

   Nonvibratory tinnitus (also called **subjective tinnitus,** because it can only be heard by the patient): Usually implies disease of the middle ear, inner ear, or eighth cranial nerve.

   Vibratory tinnitus (also called **objective tinnitus**): The conduction to the ear of sound from other structures of the head and neck, such as a vascular bruit, repetitive contraction of muscles of the palate (palatal myoclonus), or "ear popping" from the Eustachian tube.

4. What is a conductive hearing loss? A sensorineural hearing loss? How can the two be differentiated, both by history and physical findings, and with laboratory studies?

   Conductive hearing loss: Hearing loss caused by a defect in amplification and conduction of sound to the cochlea, due to a disease process involving the outer or middle ear.

   Sensorineural hearing loss: Hearing loss caused by disease in the cochlea or the auditory nerve (See Case 18 and Fig. 51.)

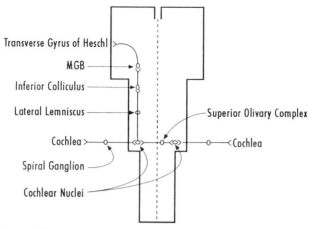

Figure 51.   Auditory pathways. MGB = medial geniculate body.

Findings/Studies	Sensorineural Hearing Loss	Conductive Hearing Loss
Type of loss	High-frequency	Low-frequency
Weber test	Lateralizes to unaffected ear	Lateralizes to affected ear
Rinne test	Air conduction > bone conduction	Bone conduction > air conduction
Audiogram	Reduced bone conduction	Normal bone conduction
	Reduced air conduction	Reduced air conduction

5. This patient felt more comfortable during her vertiginous attack when she lay on her right side. How does this fact help you to localize her lesion?

   Patients with vestibular disorders causing peripheral vertigo prefer to lie with the affected ear uppermost, because this allows them to easily look *toward* the affected side, decreasing the amount of subsequent nystagmus. Therefore, her preference to lie on the right suggests that the left labyrinth is probably affected.

6. Nystagmus with the fast-beating component to the right suggests vestibular dysfunction on which side? Why?

   Nystagmus with the fast-beating component to the right suggests dysfunction of the vestibular apparatus on the left side. The *slow* component of nystagmus beats *toward* the affected ear, and the *fast* component beats *away* from the affected ear. This occurs because lesions to the vestibular apparatus decrease the baseline rate of firing of the semicircular canals on the side of the lesion, creating a net imbalance in vestibular apparatus input into the brain-stem oculomotor system (because the unaffected semicircular canals continue to discharge at their baseline rate). The eyes, therefore, tend to drift toward the affected ear (slow component of nystagmus). The cerebral cortex subsequently provides a corrective saccade to the opposite direction (the fast component of nystagmus).

By definition, nystagmus is identified by the direction of its *fast* component. Therefore, this patient has "rightward" or "right-beating" nystagmus.

7. Given the symptom complex, what is the most likely diagnosis? What further tests would be helpful?

Diagnosis: Ménière's disease.

Further testing: ENG, audiogram.

8. How would you treat this patient?

The mainstay of therapy is conservative management with a combination of rest, antivertigo medications, acetazolamide, and salt restriction. In refractory cases with substantial baseline hearing loss, surgical treatment may be offered (endolymphatic shunting, destructive labyrinthectomy).

The Blind Beautician

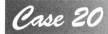

KEY TERMS

HISTORY AND EXAMINATION

History of the Present Illness

A 22-year-old right-handed beautician presents to your office with abrupt loss of vision in her right eye. She went to bed last evening without any visual complaints and awoke this morning with significant blurring in her right eye. The visual loss has continued to worsen, and she presents approximately 6 hours later.

Past Medical History

None

Medications

None

Physical Examination

P = 76/min. BP = 110/60 mm Hg. Afebrile. Head, ears, eyes, nose, and throat are normal. Lungs are clear to auscultation and percussion. Heart tones are normal, without murmurs.

Neurological Examination

In her right eye, she had light perception only. Her right optic disc was moderately swollen (Figs. 52 and 53), and a right Marcus Gunn

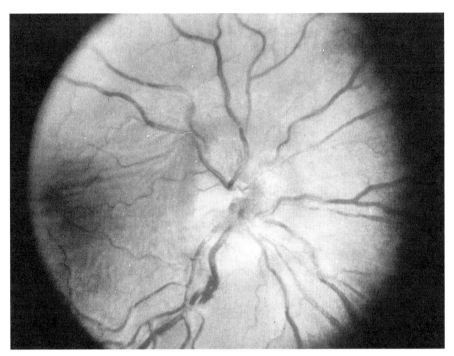

Figure 52. This fundus photo of the right optic disc reveals swelling of the optic nerve head.

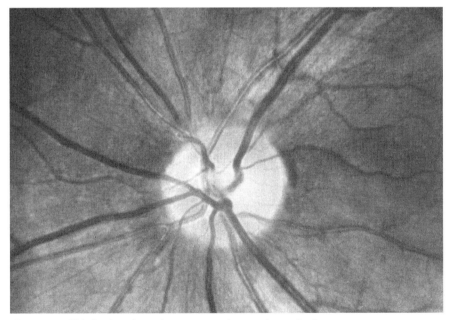

Figure 53. This fundus photo shows a normal-appearing optic disc.

pupil (an "afferent pupillary defect") was observed. (See Case 14.) The rest of the examination was normal.

CLINICAL COURSE

Her vision gradually improved over the next few months. Several months later, she again noted blurred vision. On repeat examination, when she looked to the right, one could see incomplete adduction of the left eye, with nystagmus of the right (abducting) eye. A visual evoked response (VER) was performed at that time (Fig. 54).

Two months later, she developed weakness and clumsiness of the left leg. Her examination now showed a left hemiparesis, left facial weakness, left-sided hyperreflexia, and a left Babinski's sign.

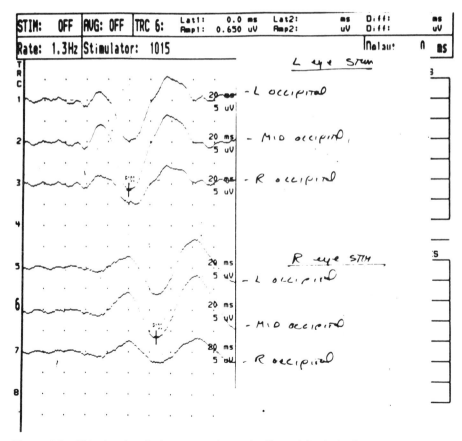

Figure 54. This visual evoked response shows significant delay in the P100 latency with right eye stimulation.

Questions

1. There are several common causes for monocular visual loss. List three, and indicate which one you think is causing this woman's problem.

2. What is a Marcus Gunn pupil? An Argyll-Robertson pupil? Describe in detail the neuroanatomic basis for each of these lesions.

3. Why was this woman's optic disc swollen? What else can cause optic disc swelling?

4. Why was this woman's vision blurred? What is an internuclear ophthalmoplegia (INO)? List two common causes for an INO.

5. Why do you think the P100 wave latency in her VER (Fig. 54) is prolonged in her right eye?

6. What is nystagmus? List five different causes for nystagmus. Why does this patient have nystagmus?

7. Facial weakness (palsy) can be due to lower or upper motor neuron lesions. How can you differentiate clinically between these two? Which type of facial palsy do you think this woman has?

8. Where is the lesion responsible for this woman's left-sided motor findings?

9. Why was her left leg clumsy?

10. What is the most likely diagnosis? How would you evaluate this patient further? What treatments can you offer her?

Answers

1. There are several common causes for monocular visual loss. List three and indicate which one you think is causing this woman's problem.

   Common causes of monocular visual loss include:
   - Cataract
   - Glaucoma
   - Retinal lesions
   - Retinal vein thrombosis
   - Ophthalmic artery occlusion
   - Optic neuritis (ischemic and demyelinating)
   - Optic nerve trauma

   Most likely, this patient has optic neuritis from demyelination, considering her age, onset of visual loss over hours (most consistent with demyelination), swelling of the optic disc (suggesting inflammation of the optic nerve, or optic neuritis), and the Marcus Gunn pupil (see below).

2. What is a Marcus Gunn pupil? An Argyll-Robertson pupil? Describe in detail the neuroanatomic basis for each of these lesions.

   Marcus Gunn pupil (Fig. 55): A pupil that constricts to light but does not maintain constriction or, paradoxically, may

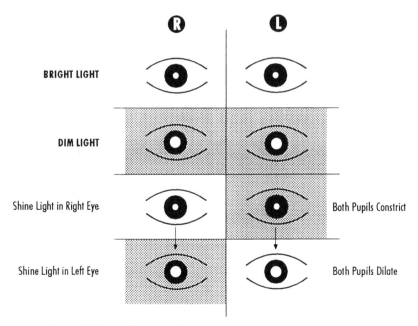

R **L**

BRIGHT LIGHT

DIM LIGHT

Shine Light in Right Eye   Both Pupils Constrict

Shine Light in Left Eye   Both Pupils Dilate

Figure 55.   Left Marcus Gunn pupil.

dilate slowly as the light continues to shine on it; the consensual reflex may be more prompt than the direct reflex (Fig. 55). These changes are best demonstrated by rapid alternate stimulation of the eyes with bright light, a technique called the "swinging flashlight test." A Marcus Gunn pupil is indicative of a lesion involving CN II.

Argyll-Robertson pupil: A pupil that does not constrict to light, although it does constrict to accommodation. This finding may be seen with syphilis involving the central nervous system, multiple sclerosis, diabetes mellitus, sarcoidosis, and alcoholic encephalopathy. An Argyll-Robertson pupil is indicative of a lesion involving the pretectum (the periaqueductal region at the level of the superior colliculus just ventral to the posterior commissure). The following figure shows pupillary light reactions, including the Argyll-Robertson pupil.

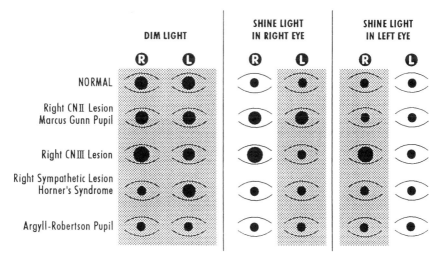

3. Why was this woman's optic disc swollen? What else can cause optic disc swelling?

Her optic disc was swollen because of inflammation of the anterior optic nerve. Optic disc swelling may be seen in two settings: with conditions that cause increased intracranial pressure (papilledema), or with conditions causing inflammation of the optic nerve (optic neuritis), such as multiple sclerosis.

Optic nerve drusen is a rare cause of optic disc swelling.

4. Why was this woman's vision blurred? What is an internuclear ophthalmoplegia (INO)? List two common causes for an INO.

Her blurred vision was due to diplopia from an INO.

Internuclear ophthalmoplegia results from a lesion of the medial longitudinal fasciculus (MLF) (Fig. 56), which results in failure of the ipsilateral eye to adduct and nystagmus of the contralateral eye with abduction. (See Case 14.)

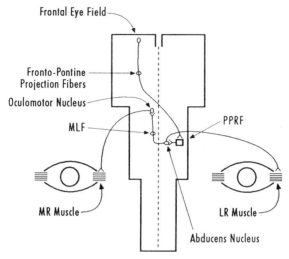

Figure 56. Cortical control of eye movements. LR Muscle = lateral rectus muscle, MR Muscle = medial rectus muscle, MLF = medial longitudinal fasciculus, PPRF = paramedian pontine reticular formation (lateral gaze center).

Causes of an INO include:
- Demyelinating lesion of the MLF
- Ischemic lesion of the MLF

5. Why do you think the P100 wave latency in her VER (Fig. 54) is prolonged in her right eye?

Her previous episode of right optic nerve demyelination (optic neuritis) has resulted in optic nerve conduction slowing. Over time, demyelinating nerve lesions frequently remyelinate, but the remyelinated segments have thinner myelin sheaths and shorter internodes. This results in slower nerve conduction velocities.

6. What is nystagmus? List five different causes for nystagmus. Why does this patient have nystagmus?

Nystagmus is an involuntary rhythmic oscillation of the eyes. Common causes include:
- Vestibular dysfunction
- Cerebellar dysfunction
- INO
- Medication (anticonvulsants)
- Congenital causes

- Physiologic causes (gaze-evoked)
- Optokinetic

This patient has nystagmus in the abducting eye because of the presence of an INO.

7. Facial weakness (palsy) can be due to lower or upper motor neuron lesions. How can you differentiate clinically between these two? Which type of facial palsy do you think this woman has?

Lower-motor neuron lesions cause weakness in both the upper and lower face, because the lesion involves the entire facial nucleus or facial nerve, which innervates one-half of the face.

Upper motor neuron (UMN) lesions cause weakness in the lower face only, because the corticobulbar tract (the UMN tract for the face) *sends both crossed and uncrossed* projections to the *upper face*, but *exclusively crossed* projections to the *lower face*. Because the upper face receives bilateral UMN innervation, it is not affected with unilateral UMN lesions (See Fig. 21, p. 63.)

This patient has UMN facial palsy because only the lower face is affected.

8. Where is the lesion responsible for this woman's left-sided motor findings?

Her left-sided motor findings are consistent with an upper motor neuron syndrome, considering hyperreflexia and Babinski's sign. Most likely these findings reflect a lesion involving the UMN tracts in the right cerebral hemisphere or brain stem.

9. Why was her left leg clumsy?

The neurological examination confirms an UMN syndrome affecting the left leg, and this is the most likely cause for the clumsiness.

10. What is the most likely diagnosis? How would you evaluate this patient further? What treatments can you offer her?

Diagnosis: Multiple sclerosis (MS). She has a separation of lesions in time (three discrete events) and space (right optic nerve, left brain stem [INO], and right upper motor neurons). (See Cases 1 and 14 for additional discussion about MS.)

Further testing: Head magnetic resonance (MR) imaging with gadolinium, to look for evidence of enhancing periventricular demyelinating lesions, which are highly suggestive of MS

Treatment:
- For symptomatic control of acute attacks: a short-term pulse of intravenous high-dose corticosteroids
- For prophylactic management to reduce the risk of subsequent attacks: interferon β-1b (Betaseron), interferon β-1a (Avonex), or glatiramer acetate (Copaxone).

The Fuzzy Lawyer

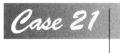

Case 21

KEY TERMS

amenorrhea: The absence or suppression of menstruation.

galactorrhea: The abnormal discharge of milk from the breasts.

visual acuity: A measure of the resolving power of the eye; usually determined by one's ability to read letters of various sizes at a standard distance from the test chart.

visual field: The area within which objects may be seen when the eye is fixed.

bitemporal hemianopia: Blindness in the temporal half of the visual field in each eye.

HISTORY AND EXAMINATION

History of the Present Illness

A 28-year-old right-handed lawyer presents to your office with progressive visual loss for the past 6 months. She first noted "fuzzy" vision in the right eye; shortly afterwards, she noted similar symptoms in the left eye. Two months ago she developed frontal and retro-orbital headaches.

Past Medical History

She has had amenorrhea of 2 years' duration, which she attributes to job-related stress.

Medications

Acetaminophen, as needed for her headache

Physical Examination

BP = 126/68 mm Hg; P = 72/min, regular. She appeared well. On general examination, her condition was normal except for the presence of galactorrhea.

Neurological Examination

Mental status is normal. Cranial nerve examination reveals pallor of the right optic disc (Fig. 57) and normal visual acuity. Visual field assessment reveals a bitemporal hemianopia. The remainder of her neurological examination is normal.

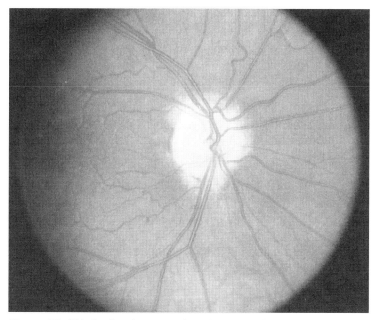

Figure 57. This fundus photo reveals optic atrophy. The optic nerve head has a "chalky-white" appearance.

Questions

1. What is bitemporal hemianopia? Draw the visual fields one would expect to see with bitemporal hemianopia. Where is the lesion that can cause this visual field defect?

2. What is homonymous hemianopia? Homonymous quadrant-anopia? Draw these visual fields and indicate where the lesions lie that cause these visual field defects.

3. What are the various ways one can test for visual field defects?

4. List three causes of bitemporal hemianopia.

5. What is amenorrhea? Galactorrhea? List several causes for these symptoms in a woman her age.

6. List five common causes for headache, and indicate what you think was the cause of this patient's headache.

7. List three causes of optic disc pallor, and indicate which one you think is involved in this case.

8. Why is her visual acuity preserved in her right eye?

9. What is the most likely diagnosis? What laboratory studies might you order? What treatment would you recommend?

10. Figure 58 shows a pathologic specimen from a patient with similar symptoms, but who died of other causes. Describe what you see. How can this lesion produce visual symptoms similar to those experienced by this patient?

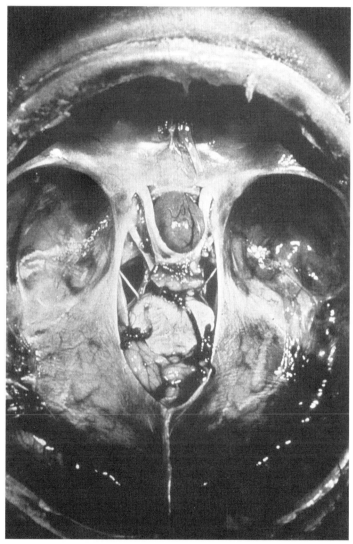

Figure 58. A gross pathologic specimen from a patient with symptoms similar to those in Case 21. This is an axial view, looking down at the base of the skull with the brain removed and the dura intact.

Answers

1. What is bitemporal hemianopia? Draw the visual fields one would expect to see with bitemporal hemianopia. Where is the lesion that can cause this visual field defect?

   Bitemporal hemianopia: Visual loss occurring in the temporal aspect of both visual fields; usually the result of involvement of the optic chiasm, situated just above the sella turcica (Fig. 59, defect No. 2).

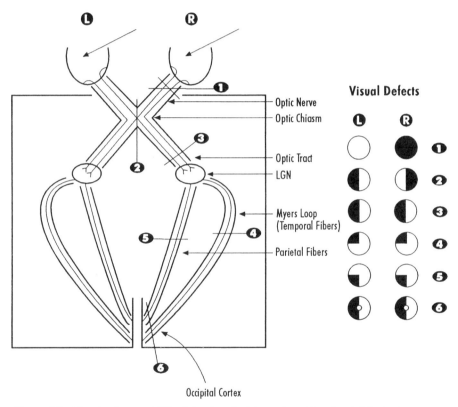

Figure 59. Visual pathways. LGN = lateral geniculate nucleus. The visual defects shown are:

Lesion Location	Visual Field Deficit
1. Right optic nerve	Right monocular blindness
2. Optic chiasm	Bitemporal hemianopia
3. Right optic tract	Left homonymous hemianopia
4. Right optic radiations (temporal fibers)	Left superior homonymous quadrantanopia
5. Right optic radiations (parietal fibers)	Left inferior homonymous quadrantanopia
6. Right visual (occipital) cortex	Left homonymous hemianopia (with macular sparing)

2. What is homonymous hemianopia? Homonymous quadrant-
   anopia? Draw these visual fields and indicate where the lesions
   lie that cause these visual field defects.

   Homonymous hemianopia: Loss of vision in the nasal half
   of the visual field in one eye and in the temporal half of the visual field in the other eye (Fig. 59, defect Nos. 3 or 6).

   Homonymous quadrantanopia: Loss of vision in the upper (or lower) nasal quadrant in one eye and in the corresponding upper or lower temporal quadrant in the other eye (Fig. 59,
   defect Nos. 4 or 5).

   Retrochiasmal lesions (lesions posterior to the optic chiasm
   and involving the optic tract, the lateral geniculate nucleus, the
   optic radiations, or the occipital cortex) may cause homonymous hemianopias or quadrantanopias.

3. What are the various ways one can test for visual field defects?

   Three ways of testing for visual field defects are:

   Confrontation testing: A routine part of the neurological
   examination during which the examiner compares the patient's
   visual fields to his or her own visual fields. In this method, the
   examiner stands directly in front of the patient, usually 2 to 3
   feet away. The patient closes one eye and looks at the examiner's nose with the other eye. The examiner does the same. A
   target (usually the examiner's finger) is then introduced from
   the periphery of each visual quadrant, and the visual field is
   assessed in this quadrant using the examiner's visual field as
   the control. Each eye is checked individually.

   Tangent screen: A formal method of measuring visual fields
   by moving a bright object against a black background screen
   into the patient's visual field.

   Goldman fields: A formal, automated method of measuring
   visual fields by using a dome of intermittently flashing bright
   lights.

4. List three causes of bitemporal hemianopia.

   Bitemporal hemianopia implies a lesion compressing the op-
   tic chiasm. Several common chiasmatic lesions producing a
   bitemporal hemianopia include:
   • Pituitary adenoma
   • Craniopharyngioma
   • Optic nerve glioma affecting the optic chiasm
   • Aneurysm compressing the optic chiasm

5. What is amenorrhea? Galactorrhea? List several causes for these symptoms in a woman her age.

   Amenorrhea: The absence or suppression of menstruation.

   Galactorrhea: The abnormal discharge of milk from the breasts.

   Possible causes for these symptoms in a young woman are:
   - Lactation (flow of milk after pregnancy while breast-feeding)
   - Prolactinoma
   - Dopamine antagonists (phenothiazines)
   - Hypothyroidism
   - Anorexia

6. List five common causes for headache, and indicate what you think was the cause of this patient's headache.

   Common causes of headache include:
   - Essential headache
     - Cluster migraines
     - Tension-type headache
   - Symptomatic headache
     - Supratentorial mass lesions (tumor, abscess, hemorrhage)
     - Meningeal irritation, due to infection (meningitis) or blood (subarachnoid hemorrhage)
     - Raised intracranial pressure (pseudotumor cerebri)
     - Pituitary mass
     - Referred pain (sinusitis, ear disease, eye disease, dental disease, cervical arthritis)

   A pituitary mass is the most likely cause of headache in this patient because she has bitemporal hemianopia, which localizes her lesion to the optic chiasm, as well as amenorrhea and galactorrhea, which suggest adenoma of the pituitary gland.

7. List three causes of optic disc pallor, and indicate which one you think is involved in this case.

   Optic disc pallor may be caused by:
   - Optic atrophy following optic neuritis
   - Optic nerve compression
   - Optic nerve ischemia
   - Glaucoma

   Compression of the optic nerve by a pituitary mass is the most likely cause of optic pallor in this patient because all other signs (bitemporal hemianopia) and symptoms (amenorrhea and galactorrhea) suggest the presence of a pituitary adenoma.

8. Why is her visual acuity preserved in her right eye?

   Visual acuity tests central vision only, which is processed by the macula. Lesions resulting in peripheral visual loss, including bitemporal and homonymous hemianopias, do not affect visual acuity. This patient has bitemporal hemianopia due to a pituitary mass, and hence her visual acuity is not affected.

9. What is the most likely diagnosis? What laboratory studies might you order? What treatment would you recommend?

   Diagnosis: Pituitary adenoma (prolactinoma).
   Further Testing:
   * Head magnetic resonance imaging (MRI) with views of the sella turcica (to visualize the pituitary mass)
   * Thyroid function tests (to rule out hypothyroidism, which may occur in conjunction with a pituitary adenoma)
   * Prolactin level (this is elevated in patients with a pituitary adenoma)
   * Follicle-stimulating hormone/luteinizing hormone (FSH/LH) levels (levels of these hormones may be low in patients with a pituitary adenoma)

   Treatment: Possible treatments for patients with pituitary adenomas include:
   * Bromocriptine (a dopamine agonist, which inhibits prolactin secretion by prolactinomas and frequently shrinks the tumor in size)
   * Surgical resection (if the tumor is large and does not decrease in size despite a trial of bromocriptine)
   * Pituitary irradiation (if surgical resection is contraindicated for any reason)

10. Figure 58 shows a pathologic specimen from a patient with similar symptoms, but who died of other causes. Describe what you see. How can this lesion produce visual symptoms similar to those experienced by this patient?

    A sellar mass (i.e., a pituitary adenoma) extends out of the sella turcica, compressing the anterior aspect of the optic chiasm.

    Because the retinal fibers that cross in the optic chiasm originate in both nasal retinae, a lesion to the optic chiasm will result in a bitemporal visual field defect because the nasal retinal fibers process temporal vision.

The Bruised Baker

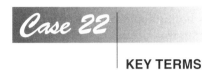

KEY TERMS

carotid bruit: A murmur heard in the cervical area that does not disappear with venous compression, is maximal over the carotid bifurcation, and is not due to transmitted cardiac murmurs.

Snellen's chart: A chart imprinted with lines of black letters graduating in size from smallest on the bottom to largest on top; used for testing distance visual acuity at a distance of 20 feet.

Jeager card: A card imprinted with lines of black letters graduating in size from smallest on the bottom to largest on top; used for testing near visual acuity at a distance of 14 inches.

atherosclerosis: The most common form of arteriosclerosis, marked by cholesterol-lipid-calcium deposits in arterial linings.

HISTORY AND EXAMINATION

History of the Present Illness

A 69-year-old, left-handed, retired baker presents to your office with the chief complaint: "I keep walking into things." During the past 7 days, she has fallen twice but luckily did not hurt herself. The falls were caused by striking furniture with her right leg while walking in her house. She has also struck her right shoulder on many occasions when walking through doorways and turning right corners. Not surprisingly, she has several bruises as proof of her recent collisions. She has a difficult time describing her vision but states that she just does not see things as clearly in her right peripheral vision. Two days before the onset of her visual problems, she experienced a 5- to 10-minute episode of diplopia without recurrence. Otherwise, she reports no weakness, numbness, or gait difficulties.

Past Medical History

Significant for hypertension (13 years) and tobacco use (more than 35 pack years). She wears bifocals.

Medications

Enalapril (an angiotensin converting enzyme [ACE] inhibitor used to treat hypertension)

Physical Examination

She is concerned about her visual complaints. P = 76/min, regular; BP = 158/91 mm Hg. Cardiac examination reveals normal heart sounds without murmurs. A faint left carotid bruit is heard.

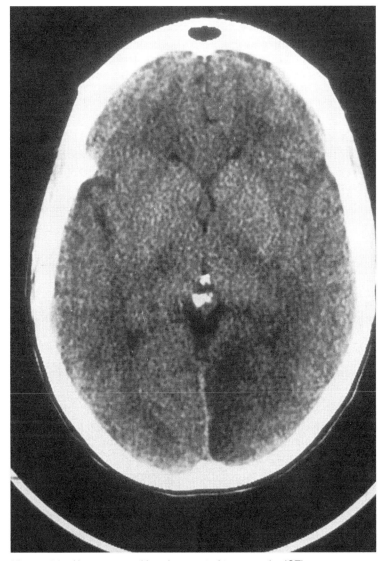

Figure 60. Noncontrasted head computed tomography (CT) scan.

Neurological Examination

Her mental status is normal. On cranial nerve testing, her visual acuity (corrected) is 20/20 with the Snellen chart and J1/J1 with the Jeager chart. Fundi reveal sharp discs and mild arteriolar narrowing. There is no afferent pupillary defect (Marcus Gunn pupil). Visual fields to confrontation reveal a right homonymous hemianopia. Ocular motility is full in all primary directions of gaze. The rest of her cranial nerves are normal. Motor, sensory, and cerebellar testing reveal no deficits. Muscle stretch reflexes are 2+ throughout, with plantar flexor responses bilaterally. Gait is normal, but she walked into the fire extinguisher that was hanging on the right side of the hallway.

You arrange for her to have a head CT scan (Fig. 60).

Questions

1. What is homonymous hemianopia? How does it differ from heteronymous hemianopia?

2. Compare the visual loss in this patient with the visual losses in the patients in Cases 20 and 21. How do these visual losses differ from one another both clinically and anatomically?

3. Why does this patient *not* have an afferent pupillary defect (Marcus Gunn pupil)?

4. What is the importance of having the patient wear her eyeglasses while checking her visual acuity?

5. Describe the abnormalities you see in her head CT scan (Fig. 60), which was obtained 10 days after her visual problems began.

6. What artery supplies the region that is affected on the CT scan?

7. What is diplopia? Why do you think the patient had diplopia? What is the generic term for transient neurological episodes?

8. Is her left carotid bruit significant?

9. What is the mechanism of disease that caused the patient's visual loss?

10. How would you manage the patient?

Answers

1. What is homonymous hemianopia? How does it differ from heteronymous hemianopia?

Hemianopia refers to loss of vision in one half of the visual field. The term homonymous indicates that visual loss is similar in both eyes, affecting either the right side of the visual field or the left side of the visual field in each eye (Fig. 61, defect No. 3, 4, 5, or 6). This patient has right homonymous hemianopia, which indicates visual loss in the right half of the visual field of each eye.

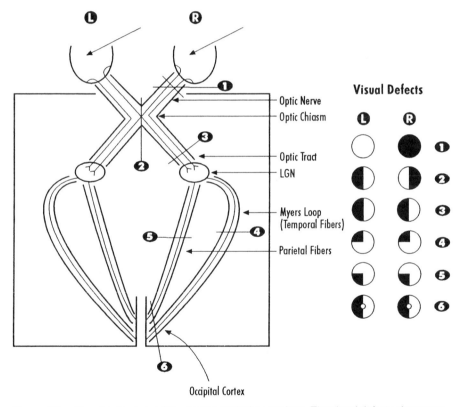

Figure 61. Visual pathways. LGN = lateral geniculate nucleus. The visual defects shown are:

Lesion Location	Visual Field Deficit
1. Right optic nerve	Right monocular blindness
2. Optic chiasm	Bitemporal hemianopia
3. Right optic tract	Left homonymous hemianopia
4. Right optic radiations (temporal fibers)	Left superior homonymous quadrantanopia
5. Right optic radiations (parietal fibers)	Left inferior homonymous quadrantanopia
6. Right visual (occipital) cortex	Left homonymous hemianopia (with macular sparing)

In heteronymous hemianopia, the pattern of visual loss in one eye involves the right visual field and in the other eye involves the left visual field. This pattern of opposite right-left visual loss can be described as *bitemporal* when the temporal field of each eye (i.e., the right half of the visual field of the right eye and the left half of the visual field of the left eye) is affected (Fig. 61, defect No. 2). The term *binasal* can be used in the opposite situation, when the left (nasal) half of the visual field of the right eye and the right (nasal) half of the visual field of the left eye are affected.

2. Compare the visual loss in this patient with the visual losses in the patients in Cases 20 and 21. How do these visual losses differ from one another both clinically and anatomically?

   In Case 20, the patient had a monocular visual loss from optic neuritis. The localization of this lesion is in the optic nerve (Fig. 61, defect No. 1). In Case 21, the patient had a heteronymous hemianopia (bitemporal visual field defect) from a chiasmal lesion caused by a pituitary adenoma (Fig. 61, defect No. 2). In the present case, the right homonymous hemianopia is localized to a lesion in the left occipital lobe (similar to Fig. 61, defect No. 6, which is a lesion in the right occipital lobe).

3. Why does this patient *not* have an afferent pupillary defect (Marcus Gunn pupil)?

   The lesion causing right homonymous hemianopia is localized to the left occipital cortex. An afferent pupillary defect is caused by a lesion to the afferent fibers of the pupillary light reflex. These afferent loop fibers never reach the occipital cortex, because they diverge toward the Edinger-Westphal nucleus in the midbrain before the optic tract reaches the lateral geniculate nucleus of the thalamus.

4. What is the importance of having the patient wear her eyeglasses while checking her visual acuity?

   By wearing glasses, one eliminates refractive errors as a cause of reduced visual acuity.

5. Describe the abnormalities you see in her head CT scan (Fig. 60), which was obtained 10 days after her visual problems began.

   This head CT scan shows an area of hypolucency (dark area) in the left occipital lobe (on the right side of the image), which is consistent with ischemic cerebral infarction. There is also calcification of the midline pineal gland, a normal finding.

6. What artery supplies the region that is affected on the CT scan?

   The blood supply to the left occipital cortex is from the left posterior cerebral artery. The right and left posterior cerebral arteries are continuation arteries from the basilar artery. The vertebral arteries, the basilar artery, and the posterior cerebral arteries, as well as their branches, are often collectively referred to as the posterior circulation.

7. What is diplopia? Why do you think the patient had diplopia? What is the generic term for transient neurological episodes?

Diplopia: The subjective sensation of seeing double (i.e., double vision). It is often caused by a brain-stem lesion that disrupts binocular control of vision. Considering that this patient had an occipital lobe ischemic infarction, it is likely that she has more diffuse cerebrovascular disease in the posterior circulation, which affects either the vertebral arteries or basilar artery.

Transient neurological deficits such as diplopia, which are caused by temporary reductions in cerebral blood flow, are called transient ischemic attacks (TIAs).

8. Is her left carotid bruit significant?

The left carotid bruit indicates that she is at risk for generalized atherosclerotic cerebrovascular disease. It does not suggest that the carotid artery was the origin of her stroke because the carotid artery subserves the anterior circulation, not the posterior circulation. The anterior circulation consists of the carotid arteries, the anterior cerebral arteries, and the middle cerebral arteries, as well as their branches.

9. What is the mechanism of disease that caused the patient's visual loss?

Most likely she has atherosclerotic vertebrobasilar disease, which caused an artery-to-artery embolus or a thrombotic occlusion. Another source of the embolus, such as the heart or aortic arch, is also possible.

10. How would you manage the patient?

Further diagnostic testing would be required. This would include an electrocardiogram to assess for underlying cardiac disease and a transesophageal echocardiogram to search for a cardiac embolus. One could also consider a head magnetic resonance angiogram, which could assess the patency or degree of athero-occlusive disease of the vertebrobasilar circulation.

In addition to maintaining adequate blood pressure control, one needs to consider either antiplatelet agents (e.g., aspirin or clopidogrel) or anticoagulants for secondary stroke prevention. The choice depends on the etiology of her stroke. If a cardiac embolus is found, strong consideration should be given to anticoagulants.

The Orthostatic Truck Driver

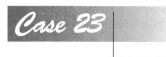

| KEY TERMS

bradykinesia: Loss of speed and spontaneity of movement.

orthostatic hypotension: A drop in blood pressure occurring when a person assumes an upright position from a supine position.

hypomimia: Loss of speed and spontaneity of facial movements.

atypical parkinsonism: A syndrome consisting of symmetrical rigidity, bradykinesia, and postural instability. It does not respond well to levodopa (L-dopa) therapy, and tremor is usually absent. Patients with idiopathic Parkinson's disease, on the other hand, typically present with resting tremor, rigidity, bradykinesia, and postural instability. The findings are usually asymmetrical, and patients respond well to L-dopa therapy.

HISTORY AND EXAMINATION

History of the Present Illness

S.D., a 65-year-old retired truck driver, was referred for a neurological opinion for multiple complaints.

Three years ago he started complaining of episodic dizziness, especially when standing up. He also noticed that his movements have become much slower. It now takes him 40 minutes to get dressed in the morning. Over the past 2 years, he has become impotent and has had problems emptying his bladder. He also complains of chronic constipation.

Past Medical History

Osteoarthritis in the knees bilaterally; appendectomy 25 years ago

Medications

Ibuprofen as needed for arthritis

Physical Examination

BP = 130/80 mm Hg supine and 95/65 mm Hg standing; P = 80/min supine; it did not change with standing.

Neurological Examination

His pupils were unequal and sluggishly reactive. There was mild symmetrical rigidity in his extremities and moderate bradykinesia. His muscle power was grade 5 in all groups; he had no tremor. His sensory examination was normal. Cerebellar examination showed mild finger-to-nose ataxia bilaterally. Muscle stretch reflexes were diffusely hyperactive. He had an extensor plantar response on the left. His gait was slightly wide-based, slow, and showed markedly diminished arm swing. He required three to four steps to recover from being gently pushed backwards.

He was started on carbidopa/levodopa (Sinemet) but showed no improvement in his walking despite large doses of medication.

Questions

1. What is the definition of orthostatic hypotension?

2. What are the common causes of orthostatic hypotension?

3. Describe the normal physiological events that come into play to minimize blood pressure changes when one assumes a standing position.

4. How is lack of a pulse rise from supine to standing helpful in differentiating primary from secondary orthostatic hypotension?

5. What other historical information indicates the presence of autonomic dysfunction in this patient?

6. What are hypomimia and bradykinesia and what is their significance?

7. What is atypical parkinsonism? What findings indicate its presence in this patient?

8. List the multiple neurological systems involved in this patient, as evidenced by his examination.

9. What is the diagnosis?

10. Where is the site of pathology?

Answers

1. What is the definition of orthostatic hypotension?

   A drop in blood pressure occurring when a person assumes an upright position from a supine position

2. What are the common causes of orthostatic hypotension?

   Secondary causes: Hypovolemia, vasodilating medications, Addison's disease.

   Primary causes: (1) Diseases affecting the peripheral autonomic nervous system, such as acute inflammatory polyneuropathy (Guillain-Barré syndrome) and diabetic and amyloid neuropathies; (2) diseases causing central autonomic dysfunction, such as progressive autonomic failure alone or with multisystem atrophy (Shy-Drager Syndrome).

3. Describe the normal physiological events that come into play to minimize blood pressure changes when one assumes a standing position.

   Standing results in pooling of blood in the veins of the lower abdomen, pelvis, and lower extremities. Venous return to the heart decreases and cardiac output drops by 10%. The resultant drop in blood pressure (BP) triggers baroreceptors in the aortic arch, carotid sinuses, and atria. The signal from the baroreceptors is relayed to the medullary vasomotor center via the afferent fibers of the glossopharyngeal nerve (cranial nerve IX) and results in increased sympathetic outflow. A concomitant decrease in vagal tone causes the heart rate to increase.

4. How is lack of a pulse rise from supine to standing helpful in differentiating primary from secondary orthostatic hypotension?

   By definition, patients with secondary orthostatic hypotension have an intact autonomic nervous system. In these patients, a systolic BP drop of 35 mm Hg would trigger a significant increase in heart rate. Therefore, the lack of a pulse rise in this patient indicates that he has primary orthostatic hypotension.

5. What other historical information indicates the presence of autonomic dysfunction in this patient?

   Impotence, urinary retention, constipation, sluggishly reactive pupils

6. What are hypomimia and bradykinesia, and what is their significance?

   Hypomimia designates diminished facial expression, whereas *bradykinesia* designates slowness of movement. Considering this patient's rigidity and postural instability, both of these findings indicate the presence of parkinsonism.

7. What is atypical parkinsonism? What findings indicate its presence in this patient?

Atypical parkinsonism is a syndrome consisting of *symmetrical* rigidity, bradykinesia, and postural instability. It does *not* respond well to carbidopa/levodopa (Sinemet) therapy. Tremor is usually *absent* in this syndrome. Patients with *idiopathic Parkinson's disease,* on the other hand, typically present with resting tremor, rigidity, bradykinesia, and postural instability. The findings are usually *asymmetrical* and respond well to Sinemet therapy.

In this patient, the absence of resting tremor, the prominent autonomic disturbances, eye movement abnormalities, cerebellar findings, and the lack of response to carbidopa/levodopa are features suggestive of atypical parkinsonism and indicate the presence of one of a group of illnesses known as the *multisystem atrophies*.

8. List the multiple neurological systems involved in this patient, as evidenced by the examination.

Autonomic nervous system, corticospinal tracts, cerebellar connections, and basal ganglia.

9. What is the diagnosis?

The presence of atypical parkinsonian features with prominent autonomic disturbance makes the *Shy-Drager syndrome* the most likely diagnosis. This degenerative illness is also described as idiopathic orthostatic hypotension with multisystem atrophy.

10. Where is the site of pathology?

In the intermediolateral cell column and dorsal vagal nuclei, where loss of cells occurs along with degeneration of the striatonigral, pyramidal, and olivopontocerebellar tracts.

The Witch's Student

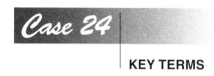

KEY TERMS

automatisms: Automatic actions or behavior without conscious volition or knowledge.

lethargy: A condition of functional torpor or sluggishness; stupor.

hirsutism: Condition characterized by the excessive growth of hair or the presence of hair in unusual places, especially in women.

aura: A subjective sensation that precedes a paroxysmal attack.

electroencephalogram (EEG): Indirect assessment of the brain's neuronal activity by recording the electrical activity from the surface of the scalp.

HISTORY AND EXAMINATION

History of the Present Illness

S.P. is a 13-year-old, left-handed girl who is referred to you by her psychiatrist for spells.

S.P. had a normal birth and childhood until she was 8 years old, when she was struck by a drunk driver while walking home from school. She lost consciousness for 15 minutes and was hospitalized for observation for 3 days. For about 6 months after the accident, S.P. complained of almost constant headaches, lethargy, and blurry vision. Her parents noted that she was more irritable, short-tempered, and could not concentrate.

Three years after the accident, S.P. began complaining of an unpleasant smell, which she described as "burning rubber" and which would last for a few minutes at a time. One morning soon thereafter, her brother found her lying on the floor "shaking all over and foaming at the mouth." Her physician diagnosed a seizure disorder and prescribed phenytoin and phenobarbital, but her family continued to notice spells of strange behavior.

About once a week thereafter, S.P. would have spells during which she described smelling "burning rubber" and would then imagine herself to be in her third grade classroom, where her teacher would be writing an arithmetic problem on the board. S.P. would raise her hand to answer the problem, but her teacher would turn into an "ugly witch" and fly at her. Family members would see S.P. wrinkle her nose during these spells, turn to her left, raise her left hand, and then turn and run. She looked sweaty and scared and her right pupil enlarged. These episodes lasted between 30 seconds and 3 minutes. After these spells, S.P. appeared scared, confused, and tired for about 30 minutes. Her left arm seemed weak, and she would not comprehend what was spoken to her. Once, during a particularly long spell, S.P. fell to the ground and her left arm shook rhythmically for 5 minutes, after which she slept for the rest of the afternoon. At times, S.P. found that she could stop a spell from continuing by repeating nursery rhymes to herself when she first smelled the "burning rubber."

School work deteriorated, particularly spelling and grammar, and teachers complained that S.P. often disrupted classes and picked fights. She began writing long essays about mysticism. The school referred her to a child psychiatrist and a speech therapist.

Past Medical History

Head trauma at age 8, as described above.

Medications

Dilantin (phenytoin) and phenobarbital

Physical Examination

Remarkable for slightly coarse facial features, mild hirsutism, and an old laceration over the right occipital area

Neurological Examination

On mental status testing, she was alert, oriented, inattentive, and restless, with decreased memory (she recalled only one of three objects after 5 minutes) and paraphasic errors. Cranial nerve testing was normal except for bilateral horizontal and vertical nystagmus. Motor examination revealed normal muscle power, tone, and bulk. She had a left pronator drift and decreased rapid alternating movements with the left hand. Sensation was normal. Her biceps and brachioradialis muscle stretch reflexes were hyperactive on the left, but all others were symmetrical, and plantar responses were flexor bilaterally. She tended to sway from side to side when walking and could not perform a tandem gait.

A head magnetic resonance (MR) scan (Fig. 62) was performed. In addition, an EEG (Fig. 63) was performed while she was not having any clinical manifestations of seizures.

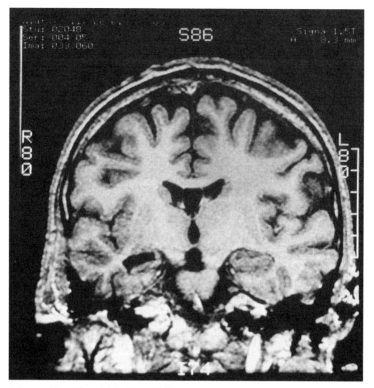

Figure 62. T1-weighted head MR scan.

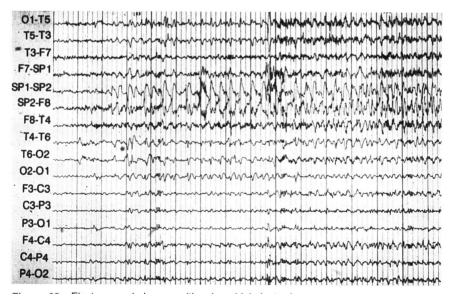

Figure 63. Electroencephalogram with sphenoidal electrodes.

Questions

1. What is a seizure? What is a convulsion? What is epilepsy? Which one does S.P. have?

2. What is the difference between a partial and a generalized seizure? Which one does S.P. have? What is a *grand mal seizure*?

3. What is the initial symptom of S.P.'s seizure? In what part of the central nervous system (CNS) does it start? Where does it spread to? What is an *aura*?

4. When rhythmic arm and leg movements were seen, what parts of the brain were being affected?

5. Describe the pathophysiology of seizures. What do you think is the cause of S.P.'s seizures?

6. What structures are being affected to cause the sweating and dilated pupil?

7. S.P.'s ataxic gait and nystagmus have developed recently. What structure is being affected? What is the cause?

8. After a seizure, S.P. experiences weakness and an inability to comprehend. Why? What is a *postictal state*?

9. Describe the abnormality present on her coronal MR scan (Fig. 62). Is the location of the abnormality similar to where you thought the initial symptoms of her seizure began?

10. What is an EEG? How does this test help in diagnosing and classifying seizures?

11. What abnormalities are present on her EEG (Fig. 63)? Does it surprise you that these abnormalities can be present even when the patient is not having symptoms?

12. Phenobarbital and phenytoin are gradually switched to another medicine, carbamazepine 200 mg twice daily. S.P. becomes more awake, more attentive, less irritable, and her grades improve. Ataxia resolves but nystagmus continues. The seizures also decrease, so that she only has the sensation of burning rubber once a month without other symptoms. What should you do now?

13. In 2 years, S.P. will want to learn to drive. What will you tell her? What advice would you give her about how long she should continue taking the medication?

Answers

1. What is a seizure? What is a convulsion? What is epilepsy? Which one does S.P. have?

   Seizure: A cortical electrical discharge producing a neurological symptom or sign.

   Convulsion: A seizure associated with motor activity.

   Epilepsy: A chronic neurological disorder manifested by recurrent seizures.

   S.P. has all three.

2. What is the difference between a partial and a generalized seizure? Which one does S.P. have? What is a *grand mal seizure*?

   Partial (focal) seizure: A seizure limited to a single focal area of brain; consciousness is typically preserved. The symptoms of a partial seizure reflect the part of the brain that is discharging (e.g., a seizure coming from the motor cortex will result in a convulsion). Partial seizures may be *simple partial* (consciousness is fully preserved) or *complex partial* (consciousness is altered but not lost entirely). Complex partial seizures usually involve large areas of parietal and temporal association cortex and produce complex symptomatology. For example, S.P. wrinkled her nose, turned to her left, raised her left hand, and then turned and ran. Such complex, repetitive behaviors are termed automatisms.

   Generalized seizure: A seizure involving both hemispheres; consciousness is lost. Generalized seizures may be *primarily generalized* (involving both hemispheres from the start of the seizure) or *secondarily generalized* (beginning focally, then spreading through the corpus callosum to involve both hemispheres).

   S.P. is having complex partial and secondarily generalized seizures.

   Grand mal seizure is an old term for a generalized motor seizure.

3. What is the initial symptom of S.P.'s seizure? In what part of the CNS does the seizure start? Where does it spread to? What is an *aura*?

   The initial symptom of S.P.'s seizures is smelling burning rubber.

   The seizure starts in the uncus and spreads to the temporal lobe.

An *aura* is a simple partial seizure without motor movements; it is usually the initial symptom of a complex partial seizure.

4. When rhythmic arm and leg movements were seen, what parts of the brain were being affected?

The contralateral motor cortex.

5. Describe the pathophysiology of seizures. What do you think is the cause of S.P.'s seizures?

A seizure represents an abnormal electrical discharge of the brain, usually arising from an area of injured cortex.

S.P.'s seizures are probably due to a cortical scar from her past head trauma.

6. What structures are being affected to cause the sweating and dilated pupil?

The seizure spreads to involve the hypothalamus, the head nucleus for the sympathetic nervous system. The seizure causes excitation of the hypothalamus, thereby increasing sympathetic outflow. Both sweating and pupillary dilatation are symptoms of increased sympathetic activity.

7. S.P.'s ataxic gait and nystagmus have developed recently. What structure is being affected? What is the cause?

Symptoms of gait ataxia and nystagmus can be due to dysfunction of the cerebellum. The most common side effects associated with elevated serum levels of phenytoin are nystagmus and gait ataxia; both are thought to be due to drug-related cerebellar toxicity. When the dosage of phenytoin (and hence, the serum level) is lowered, these symptoms will be reversed.

8. After a seizure, S.P. experiences weakness and an inability to comprehend. Why? What is a *postictal state*?

S.P.'s deficits are caused by depletion of substrates (glucose) from areas of the brain that are actively discharging during the seizure (*Todd's paralysis*).

A *postictal state* is a period of disorientation and fatigue (and occasionally focal weakness) that follows a seizure. The postictal state commonly lasts for hours and may last up to a day or two, depending on the severity of the seizure.

9. Describe the abnormality present on her coronal MR scan (Fig. 62). Is the location of the abnormality similar to where you thought the initial symptoms of her seizure began?

The head MR scan reveals right hippocampal atrophy and compensatory dilatation of the right temporal horn of the lateral ventricle. Also note the generalized cortical atrophy with widening of the cortical sulci.

Focal seizures often begin in areas where there is preexisting injury. In addition, the temporal lobe is the area in the brain that is most prone to the development of focal seizures.

10. What is an EEG? How does this test help in diagnosing and classifying seizures?

An EEG is a recording of cortical electrical activity from the surface of the scalp. Most of the activity recorded in the EEG consists of extracellular current flow associated with summated postsynaptic potentials in synchronously active pyramidal cells of the cerebral cortex.

Different seizure types produce different EEG patterns. A localized discharge on the EEG helps identify the seizure focus.

11. What abnormalities are present on her EEG (Fig. 63)? Does it surprise you that these abnormalities can be present even when the patient is not having symptoms?

Focal spikes representing electrical cortical discharges are emanating from the right anterior temporal lobe of the brain.

It is common to have electrical seizure activity, as evidenced by spike discharges on EEG, without any clinical manifestations of seizure activity.

12. Phenobarbital and phenytoin are gradually switched to another medicine, carbamazepine 200 mg twice daily. S.P. becomes more awake, more attentive, less irritable, and her grades improve. The ataxia resolves but the nystagmus continues. The seizures also decrease, so that she only has the sensation of burning rubber once a month without other symptoms. What should you do now?

Increase carbamazepine to achieve high therapeutic levels or until the seizures stop. Monitor the complete blood count and serum sodium, because carbamazepine may cause neutropenia and hyponatremia.

13. In 2 years, S.P. will want to learn to drive. What will you tell her? What advice would you give her about how long she should continue taking the medication?

If the patient remains seizure-free for at least 1 year on a stable therapeutic regimen, driving is permissible in most states. She should take carbamazepine indefinitely if she is having auras.

If her auras and seizures continue despite trials of antiepileptic medications, she should be referred to a comprehensive epilepsy program for consideration of surgery to remove the seizure focus.

The Absent Student

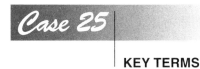

staring spells: A temporary alteration of consciousness or awareness that can result from a partial seizure, presyncope, or daydreaming.

hyperventilation: Increased minute volume ventilation that results in a lowered carbon dioxide level (hypocapnia).

HISTORY AND EXAMINATION

History of the Present Illness

Jennifer is 6-year-old, right-handed first-grade student in an accelerated learning program in an elite suburban school district. Her parents are concerned about recent changes in her behavior.

When preschool testing revealed an IQ of 145, Jennifer was enrolled in first grade last fall and had done very well up until Christmas. In January, her teacher noticed that Jennifer seemed distractible and did not grasp new material as easily as she had previously. The decreased performance level was initially attributed to the death of a grandfather shortly after Christmas. Her grades deteriorated and by March, it was suggested that Jennifer be placed in a regular class the following year. The suggestion upset her parents considerably.

Jennifer's parents began noticing brief staring spells in March. Spells would occur while Jennifer played, watched television, or read. They consisted of staring blankly for 3 to 10 seconds. During this time, Jennifer would not seem to be aware of the environment. Occasionally, she would respond to a question but much more slowly than usual. Some eye fluttering could be seen toward the end of some of the longer spells. Immediately afterward, Jennifer would resume her normal activity. For example, if she happened to be eating when a spell occurred, she might pause with a fork of spaghetti poised in midair, stare for a few seconds, and then proceed to put the spaghetti into her mouth. She did not fall, become incontinent, or have any other movements. These spells increased, and by April they occurred three times an hour. Jennifer was unaware of these spells and denied any warning symptoms.

Past Medical History

Her mother was a 27-year-old primigravida at the time of Jennifer's birth. Pregnancy, labor, and delivery were normal; no perinatal problems; usual childhood diseases; no head trauma.

Medications

None

Physical Examination

Entirely normal for age

Neurological Examination

Entirely normal for age; no spells were observed. When asked to take deep, rapid breaths, Jennifer complied. After performing well for 45 seconds, she abruptly paused, stared for 5 seconds, and then resumed deep breathing. A similar 8-second episode occurred 20 seconds later.

An electroencephalogram (EEG) was obtained (Fig. 64). Ethosuximide was prescribed. Within 2 weeks, her parents noticed a decrease in the number of staring spells. One month later, all the spells have stopped, schoolwork has returned to baseline, and Jennifer's parents are negotiating with the school to keep her in the accelerated class.

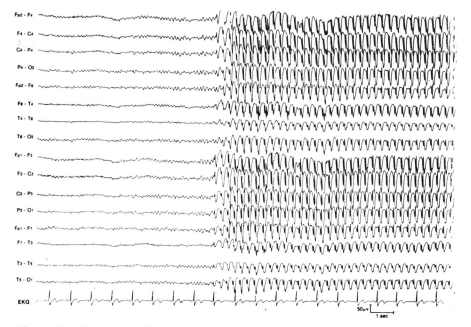

Figure 64. Electroencephalogram.

Questions

1. Does Jennifer have epilepsy? If so, what type of epilepsy does she have?

2. What is the pathophysiology of absence seizures? Are they focal or generalized seizures? How do they differ from the type of seizures exhibited by the patient in Case 24?

3. Why did hyperventilation cause Jennifer to have a seizure?

4. How would you explain the absence of any warning signs before Jennifer loses consciousness?

5. If Jennifer at most got staring spells three times per hour for less than 10 seconds at a time, why was she having so much trouble with schoolwork?

6. What is the characteristic finding seen on Jennifer's EEG (Fig. 64)? How does it differ from the EEG of S.P. in Case 24?

7. Would you order a head computed tomography (CT) scan? Magnetic resonance (MR) scan? If so, why?

8. How do you explain the fact that these seizures did not begin earlier—for example, when Jennifer was 2 years old?

9. How long will they continue? Is Jennifer likely to require medication indefinitely?

10. What would you suggest to Jennifer's parents regarding any special precautions they need to take?

Answers

1. Does Jennifer have epilepsy? If so, what type of epilepsy does she have?

   Yes, she has absence epilepsy.

2. What is the pathophysiology of absence seizures? Are they focal or generalized seizures? How do they differ from the type of seizures exhibited by the patient in Case 24?

   Absence seizures are subcortical, *centrencephalic* seizures that are thought to originate in the brain-stem reticular formation or intralaminar thalamic nuclei.

   Absence seizures are *primary generalized* seizures that do not have a focal onset.

   The patient in Case 24 was an example of a *focal* seizure disorder.

3. Why did hyperventilation cause Jennifer to have a seizure?

   Absence seizures are commonly precipitated by hyperventilation because the resultant hypocapnea activates thalamocortical pathways.

4. How would you explain the absence of any warning signs before Jennifer loses consciousness?

   Absence seizures are generalized from the outset and have an abrupt onset without an *aura*. Only partial seizures can start with an aura.

5. If Jennifer at most got staring spells three times an hour for less than 10 seconds at a time, why was she having so much trouble with schoolwork?

   She is probably having frequent subclinical seizures that interrupt her train of thought and concentration.

6. What is the characteristic finding seen on Jennifer's EEG (Fig. 64)? How does it differ from the EEG of S.P. in Case 24?

   Jennifer's EEG shows generalized, synchronized, three-per-second spike-and-wave discharges, the classic pattern seen in absence epilepsy.

   Jennifer's EEG is that of a *generalized* epilepsy; S.P.'s EEG is that of a *partial* (localization-related, focal) epilepsy.

7. Would you order a head CT scan? An MR scan? If so, why?

   Neither. There is no need for an imaging study in this patient because absence seizures are not associated with structural brain disease, such as tumors.

8. How do you explain the fact that these seizures did not begin earlier—for example, when Jennifer was 2 years old?

Absence epilepsy begins at about the age of 4 or later. It is an age-locked phenomenon that depends on the level of maturation of the brain.

9. How long will the seizures continue? Is Jennifer likely to require medication indefinitely?

Absence seizures typically resolve by the mid-to-late teenage years.

Because she will "outgrow" her seizures by the time she is a teenager, she will not require medication indefinitely.

10. What would you suggest to Jennifer's parents regarding any special precautions they need to take?

Common-sense avoidance of danger (e.g., she should not swim alone and should take showers instead of baths).

The Gopher Hunter

Case 26

KEY TERMS

orientation: The ability to comprehend and to adjust oneself in an environment with regard to time, location, and identity of persons.

paraphasia: The misuse of spoken words or word combinations; a form of aphasia.

anomia: Inability to remember names of objects.

perseveration: Continued repetition of a word or phrase, or repetition of answers that are not related to successive questions asked.

motor impersistence: Inability to sustain voluntary motor acts that have been initiated on verbal command; seen in patients with bihemispheric disease or other brain-damaged states.

paratonic rigidity: A type of alteration in the muscle tone in which the tone appears increased owing to an inability to relax the muscle. This type of rigidity is seen with bihemispheric lesions.

frontal release signs: Reflexes that are present in infancy, lost with maturation of the central nervous system, and regained with advanced age or with diffuse cortical or bihemispheric dysfunction, such as can be seen with Alzheimer's disease, Parkinson's disease, or bihemispheric strokes.

HISTORY AND EXAMINATION

History of the Present Illness

E.K. is a 68-year-old, right-handed retired senior executive of a major corporation who is referred to a neurologist because of recent unusual behavior.

E.K. was born in 1930 in Davenport, Iowa. After completing high school, he received a BS in chemistry from Iowa State University in 1951. He married his high school sweetheart in 1952 and served as a laboratory technician in the Army during the later days of the Korean War. After the war, he received a PhD in chemistry from the University of Chicago in 1959 and was offered a position in a major corporation doing research. He and his wife moved to upstate New York in 1960 along with their two children. In 1968, E.K. was promoted to a supervisory position and in 1979, was named a vice president for research. In 1992, E.K. stepped down as an executive during a major corporate reorganization. He remained affiliated with the company as a consultant until 1994, when he decided he was not interested in working.

About the time of his retirement, Mrs. K. noticed a change in E.K. He became somewhat short-tempered and gruff. He tended to forget symphony concerts and other appointments, saying, "I'm retired. I'm through with schedules." He spent increasing time watching television, gave up his hobby of collecting baseball cards, and was no longer interested in socializing ("I've had to socialize all my life. Now that I've retired, I'm going to relax"). E.K. continued to golf avidly, maintaining his lifelong average of 84. He napped frequently during the day.

By 1997, E.K. was spending all his time at home watching television or reading, except for doing odd jobs around the house, golfing, and attending baseball games. Toward the end of the baseball season, he got lost following one of the games and called Mrs. K. from a distant suburb. He decided not to go to Florida this past winter. He no longer paid close attention to grooming his hair and mustache.

Last Saturday morning, Mrs. K. heard a shotgun blast. Running to the study, she found E.K. sitting at an open window with his shotgun. He said he had seen gophers on the lawn and shot them. Shortly afterwards, the neighbor's son arrived saying that he had been mowing the lawn next door and had heard the shot whistle past his head.

E.K. had long insisted that he felt fine and didn't need to see a physician but agreed his eyesight might be failing following the gopher incident.

Past Medical History

Unremarkable. The patient is a nonsmoker. He drinks alcohol socially.

Medications

None

Physical Examination

Unremarkable

Neurological Examination

He was alert, well dressed, polite, and jocular. He was oriented to "physician's office" but could not give the day, date, or month. He said it was 1978 (it was actually 1998) and could not relate recent events. "The election is going on, but I'm not interested in all that *polemical* stuff." He could not comment on the "*basebell*" season. His speech was fluent, but he could not name various objects when they were described (e.g., when asked for the type of house Eskimos live in, he replied, "Teepee.") When asked to list 10 fruits, he said, "Apples, oranges, uh, tomatoes, potatoes, cabbage, uh, how many is that?" When asked to locate New York City on a blank map of the United States, he pointed to Peoria. When asked to count backwards from 100 by 7s, he said, "100, 93, 86, 76, 66, 56." When asked to remember three objects (tuxedo, Washington, and paper clip), his response after 5 minutes was, "Was it apples? Apples and something about ball." He was able to recall in great detail his wartime service in Korea.

The rest of the neurological examination was normal except for motor impersistence in eye movements, paratonic muscle rigidity, and the presence of snout, glabellar, palmomental, and grasp reflexes.

As part of his work-up, E.K. had a head computed tomography (CT) scan (Fig. 65).

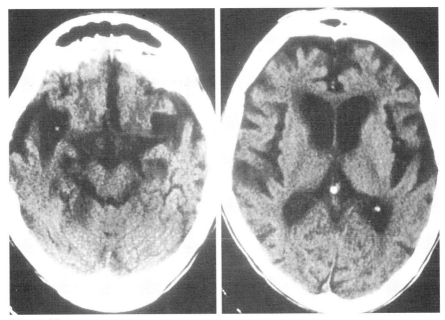

Figure 65. Head CT scan, performed without contrast.

Questions

1. What is the course of E.K.'s illness? How far back can you trace the symptoms?

2. What type of disturbance is there in his memory? Where does memory reside in the brain? What is association cortex, and what role does it play in brain function?

3. Is there any evidence of left hemispheric cortical dysfunction? Right hemispheric cortical dysfunction? Bihemispheric dysfunction?

4. Is this patient aphasic? If so, is his aphasia fluent or nonfluent? How do you decide? How does one test for aphasia?

5. What is apraxia? Agnosia? List three common examples of each.

6. What is paratonic rigidity, and with which pathologic states is it associated?

7. What is the significance of *frontal release signs* (snout, glabellar, palmomental, and grasp reflexes), and with which pathologic states are they associated?

8. Figure 65 shows E.K.'s head CT scan. What do you notice?

9. What disease processes could account for E.K.'s signs and symptoms? Could all of E.K.'s symptoms be due to depression? What is the most likely diagnosis?

10. What laboratory tests, if any, are needed? What might you expect them to show?

11. If E.K.'s aim had been better and he had hit his neighbor, how would you testify in court as to his competency to stand trial? On what grounds?

12. What advice would you have for Mrs. K?

Answers

1. What is the course of E.K.'s illness? How far back can you trace the symptoms?

   His illness is slowly progressive. It probably began in 1992, 6 years prior to his presentation, when he stepped down from his position as a vice president for research.

2. What type of disturbance is there in his memory? Where does memory reside in the brain? What is association cortex, and what role does it play in brain function?

   He primarily has a problem with short-term memory. Memory resides in diffuse areas of the cerebral cortex. Various types of memory reside in different areas of the brain. For example, short-term memory resides in the hippocampus. New information is incorporated into the hippocampus via the Papez circuit: hippocampus → fornix → mammillary bodies → mammillothalamic tract → anterior nucleus of the thalamus → cingulate cortex → hippocampus. Therefore, any lesion along the path of the Papez circuit would manifest itself as short-term memory loss.

   Long-term memory resides in association cortex. Association cortex includes large areas of the parietal, temporal, occipital, and frontal lobes that associate and integrate primary motor, sensory, visual, and auditory modalities. This integrative function also includes the storage of long-term information.

3. Is there any evidence of left hemispheric cortical dysfunction? Right hemispheric cortical dysfunction? Bihemispheric dysfunction?

   There is evidence of all these types of dysfunction:
   Left hemisphere dysfunction: aphasia, acalculia
   Right hemisphere dysfunction: geographic disorientation
   Bihemispheric dysfunction: impaired memory and cognitive function

4. Is this patient aphasic? If so, is his aphasia fluent or nonfluent? How do you decide? How does one test for aphasia?

   Yes, he has a fluent aphasia because his speech is fluent but contains many paraphasic errors.

   The aphasia examination has six components: spontaneous speech, naming, comprehension, repetition, reading, and writing.

5. What is apraxia? Agnosia? List three common examples of each.

   Apraxia: The inability to perform tasks or activities in the presence of preserved motor, sensory, and cerebellar functions (e.g., dressing, gait, grooming).

   Agnosia: The inability to recognize familiar or common environmental stimuli in the presence of preserved motor, sensory, and cerebellar functions (e.g., colors, faces, body parts).

6. What is paratonic rigidity and with which pathologic states is it associated?

   Paratonic rigidity (paratonia): The inability to relax a limb when it is passively moved. There are two types of paratonia:

   Gegenhalten: The patient moves the limb against the examiner.

   Mitgehen: The patient moves the limb with the examiner.

   Paratonia is associated with diffuse forebrain dysfunction, such as Alzheimer's disease and bihemispheric strokes.

7. What is the significance of *frontal release signs* (snout, glabellar, palmomental, and grasp reflexes), and with which pathologic states are they associated?

   Frontal release signs suggest diffuse forebrain dysfunction; they are typically seen in Alzheimer's disease and in bihemispheric strokes.

8. Figure 65 shows E.K.'s head CT scan. What do you notice?

   The CT scan shows generalized cerebral atrophy with widening of the cortical sulci and enlargement of the ventricular system. It does not offer any evidence for past cerebral infarctions, which would occur in patients with vascular dementia.

9. What disease processes could account for E.K.'s signs and symptoms? Could all of E.K.'s symptoms be due to depression? What is the most likely diagnosis?

   E.K. has a dementia, which is defined as significant loss of cognitive function involving multiple cognitive domains and not due to an impaired level of consciousness. Alzheimer's disease is the most common form of dementia in the United States, accounting for over 50% of all cases. Vascular dementia accounts for about 25%. There are many other less common causes of dementia, including Parkinson's disease, Huntington's disease, and head trauma. The progressive nature of E.K.'s symptoms and the absence of other neurological symptoms (e.g., parkinsonism or chorea) strongly suggests the diagnosis of Alzheimer's disease. Vascular dementia often presents in a stepwise fashion as a result of successive strokes.

Although depression at times mimics dementia in the elderly, E.K. has a severely impaired mental status and a fluent aphasia, which makes depression as the sole diagnosis quite unlikely.

10. What laboratory tests, if any, are needed? What might you expect them to show?

Tests for thyroid function, serum vitamin B_{12} level, syphilis serology, and chemistry and hematology profiles should be performed to rule out reversible causes of dementia. All these test results should be normal in Alzheimer's disease.

11. If E.K.'s aim had been better and he had hit his neighbor, how would you testify in court as to his competency to stand trial? On what grounds?

He is incompetent to stand trial because of dementia.

12. What advice would you have for Mrs. K?

Remove the shotgun.

Frequently reorient the patient.

Keep him in familiar surroundings.

Avoid sedative or psychoactive drugs unless he is agitated or delusional.

Contact the local Alzheimer's Association for education and support.

The Confabulating Woman

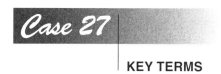

KEY TERMS

confabulation: A behavioral reaction to memory loss in which the patient fills in memory gaps with inappropriate words.

dysconjugate gaze: Disruption of coordinated and conjugate eye movements that normally maintain the visual axis of the two eyes in parallel. Dysconjugate gaze implies and can result from deep sleep or diseases of the muscle, cranial nerves, or brain stem.

heel-to-shin testing: A test of leg coordination in which the heel of one leg is run smoothly down the other shin, and speed, accuracy, and any tremor are noted.

HISTORY AND EXAMINATION

History of the Present Illness

A disheveled, emaciated woman, smelling of alcohol and appearing to be in her mid-fifties, wandered into the emergency department on Christmas Eve. Although she had no specific complaints, she could not provide any pertinent personal information aside from her name. When initially evaluated by the emergency department nurse, the patient was unable to provide her address, age, or the date. When asked what holiday was approaching, she stated "Memorial Day" even though she was dressed in warm winter garb. When asked where she was, she was initially uncertain. After taking in her environs, she decided she was in a hospital but could not provide the name or city. After each of these inquiries, she was informed of the correct answer and was able to repeat it back to the nurse. However, on requestioning 5 minutes later, it was clear that she had not retained any of the information, and in fact, she denied having seen the nurse previously. Because of these bizarre deficits, the nurse asked the intern to see the patient. The intern found that despite her disorientation, the patient was able to read, write, perform simple calculations, interpret proverbs, and even repeat a six-digit span. Baffled by this mental status examination, the intern asked for a neurology consultation. While waiting for the neurology resident, the nurse gave the patient a "holiday" meal tray filled with "goodies," which she devoured voraciously.

Past Medical History
Unknown

Medications
Unknown

Physical Examination
When the neurology resident arrived 45 minutes later, her BP = 146/84 mmHg; P = 96/min and regular.

Neurological Examination
The patient was drowsy but arousable. She claimed that it was Christmas 1970 and thought the examiner was her boyfriend of 30 years ago. She had nystagmus in all directions of gaze and had slight dysconjugate gaze when she looked to the right or left. Her muscle strength was normal. The sensory examination was notable for diminution of vibration and proprioception in her feet. She had normal finger-to-nose testing but was ataxic with heel-to-shin testing bilaterally. Her reflexes were 2+ with the exception of her ankle jerks, which were trace. She had bilateral Babinski's signs. When attempting to walk, she became quite unsteady on her feet and had a wide-based, swaying stance.

Both the nurse and the intern confirmed that her abnormal eye movements and gait abnormalities were not present initially. The absence of these abnormalities suggested to them an acute posterior fossa event that necessitated an emergent computed tomography (CT) scan. However, the neurology resident insisted on medical treatment before the CT scan.

Questions

1. How would you characterize the patient's deficits on presentation?

2. What lesion(s) might produce this pattern of abnormal memory? What particular disease entities?

3. Are there any further historical or laboratory data you would like to have on this patient?

4. What is the significance of the patient's eye movement and gait abnormalities?

5. Why did this patient's condition worsen after eating?

6. What is the most likely diagnosis in this patient? Could this be Alzheimer's disease?

7. What is the emergency treatment recommended by the neurology resident? Why? What is the prognosis for this patient?

8. Figure 66 shows a pathologic specimen from a patient who died from this condition. What does it reveal, and how can this finding cause a memory disorder?

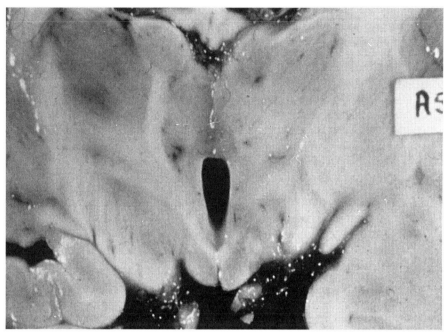

Figure 66. Gross brain specimen from a patient who died from the condition affecting The Confabulating Woman.

Answers

1. How would you characterize the patient's deficits on presentation?
   She primarily had a short-term memory deficit with frequent confabulation.

2. What lesion(s) might produce this pattern of abnormal memory? What particular disease entities?
   Bilateral lesions involving any of the components of the Papez circuit: hippocampi, mammillary bodies, anterior thalamic nuclei, and cingulate gyrus.
   Wernicke-Korsakoff syndrome (due to thiamine deficiency from alcoholism) and transient global amnesia may produce this picture.

3. Are there any further historical or laboratory data you would like to have on this patient?

Because vitamin B_{12} deficiency may cause memory impairment and neurological signs, it would be helpful to obtain a nutritional history, as well as a vitamin B_{12} level and mean corpuscular volume (MCV). (MCV elevations may indicate vitamin B_{12} deficiency.)

4. What is the significance of the patient's eye movement and gait abnormalities?

These findings represent acute Wernicke's encephalopathy, which is a clinical triad consisting of ophthalmoplegia, ataxia, and mental status abnormalities due to acute thiamine deficiency. Alcoholism may also cause peripheral neuropathy and cerebellar atrophy, both of which may result in gait abnormalities.

5. Why did this patient's condition worsen after eating?

The metabolism of glucose requires thiamine. In patients with an underlying thiamine deficiency, as in this case, ingestion of large carbohydrate loads further depletes brain thiamine concentrations and results in an acute Wernicke's encephalopathy.

6. What is the most likely diagnosis in this patient? Could this be Alzheimer's disease?

The most likely diagnosis is Wernicke-Korsakoff syndrome secondary to thiamine deficiency.

This is not Alzheimer's disease. The patient's major abnormality in mental status is in short-term memory only.

7. What is the emergency treatment recommended by the neurology resident? Why? What is the prognosis for this patient?

Emergent treatment: Intravenous thiamine, because the symptomatology of Wernicke-Korsakoff syndrome is due to a biochemical abnormality as a result of thiamine deficiency.

Prognosis: A mortality rate of 100% if not treated; 10% mortality rate in treated patients. Ophthalmoplegia resolves with treatment. Nystagmus and ataxia may persist in 35% of treated patients. Global confusion resolves with treatment, but short-term memory loss (also known as Korsakoff amnesia) persists in more than 80% of treated patients.

8. Figure 66 shows a pathologic specimen from a patient who died from this condition. What does it reveal, and how can this finding cause a memory disorder?

The mammillary bodies in this pathologic specimen are atrophic and discolored brown due to microhemorrhages.

The mammillary bodies are part of the Papez circuit, which is important in incorporating new memory (Fig. 67).

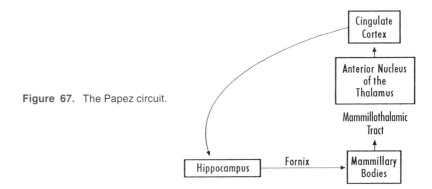

Figure 67. The Papez circuit.

Index

An "f" following a number indicates a figure.